EDITED BY
MORTEN SKOVDAL AND
LENA SKOVGAARD ANDERSEN

WITH A FOREWORD BY
SANTINO SEVERONI

CONTINUITY OF CARE FOR FORCIBLY DISPLACED PERSONS LIVING WITH CHRONIC ILLNESS

POLICY PRESS SHORTS POLICY & PRACTICE

First published in Great Britain in 2026 by

Policy Press, an imprint of
Bristol University Press
University of Bristol
1-9 Old Park Hill
Bristol
BS2 8BB
UK
t: +44 (0)117 374 6645
e: bup-info@bristol.ac.uk

Details of international sales and distribution partners are available at
policy.bristoluniversitypress.co.uk

© Morten Skovdal and Lena Skovgaard Andersen 2026

DOI: 10.51952/9781447377276

The digital PDF and ePub versions of this title are available open access and distributed under the terms of the Creative Commons Attribution-NonCommercial-NoDerivatives 4.0 International licence (https://creativecommons.org/licenses/by-nc-nd/4.0/) which permits reproduction and distribution for non-commercial use without further permission provided the original work is attributed.

British Library Cataloguing in Publication Data
A catalogue record for this book is available from the British Library

ISBN 978-1-4473-7725-2 paperback
ISBN 978-1-4473-7726-9 ePub
ISBN 978-1-4473-7727-6 OA PDF

The right of Morten Skovdal and Lena Skovgaard Andersen to be identified as editors of this work has been asserted by them in accordance with the Copyright, Designs and Patents Act 1988.

All rights reserved: no part of this publication may be reproduced, stored in a retrieval system, or transmitted in any form or by any means, electronic, mechanical, photocopying, recording, or otherwise without the prior permission of Bristol University Press.

Every reasonable effort has been made to obtain permission to reproduce copyrighted material. If, however, anyone knows of an oversight, please contact the publisher.

The statements and opinions contained within this publication are solely those of the editors and contributors and not of the University of Bristol or Bristol University Press. The University of Bristol and Bristol University Press disclaim responsibility for any injury to persons or property resulting from any material published in this publication.

Bristol University Press and Policy Press work to counter discrimination on grounds of gender, race, disability, age and sexuality.

Cover design: Chris Wilson
Front cover image: iStock/Claudiad

Contents

Notes on contributors		v
Acknowledgements		xi
Foreword		xii
one	Working holistically: dimensions shaping continuity of care for forcibly displaced persons living with chronic illness *Morten Skovdal, Saria Hassan, Johanna Hanefeld, and Lena Skovgaard Andersen*	1
PART I	**Navigational capacity**	
two	Working with perceptions: patient education and counselling as pathways to continuity of care among diabetic patients in Gaza *Usama Lubbad*	15
three	Working with agency: agency as a driver of continuity of HIV care among Ukrainian refugees fleeing to Denmark *Emilie Mai Anderberg, Marie Nørredam, and Morten Skovdal*	37
PART II	**Social relations**	
four	Working through community structures: the role of community health workers in cardio-metabolic disease care in Bidibidi, Uganda *Tania Aase Dræbel, Bishal Gyawali, Dricile Ratib, Rita Nakanjako, Esther Kalule Nanfuka, Emmanuel Raju, David Kyanddodo, and Morten Skovdal*	57

five	Working alongside interpreters: optimising communication for continuity of care for refugees in Uganda	78
	Rita Nakanjako, Esther Kalule Nanfuka, Morten Skovdal, Susan Reynolds Whyte, and David Kyaddondo	

PART III Programmatic organisation

six	Working for access: how Red Cross in Georgia works to ensure diagnostics and continuity of HIV care and treatment for Ukrainian refugees	103
	Davron Mukhamadiev, Nana Tsanava, and Tea Chikviladze	
seven	Working with mental health: how integrating mental health and psychosocial support into refugee health services can support continuity of care for chronic conditions	118
	Ye Htut Oo	
eight	Working across sectors: how multi-sectoral integration improves participation in mental health and psychosocial support interventions for refugees	135
	Jacqueline Ntombizodwa Ndlovu	
nine	Working towards continuity of care: calls for action for forcibly displaced persons living with chronic illness	153
	Lena Skovgaard Andersen and Morten Skovdal	

Index 156

Notes on contributors

Emilie Mai Anderberg is a global health specialist dedicated to advancing health equity and strengthening sustainable health systems. Drawing on experience across low- and middle-income countries, she applies intersectional and community-driven approaches to address structural inequities. Her work centres on the lived experiences of marginalised and underserved communities, ensuring these inform inclusive policies and equitable access to care.

Lena Skovgaard Andersen is Associate Professor of Global Mental Health at the University of Copenhagen and Director of its School of Global Health. She also holds an honorary position in the HIV Mental Health Research Unit at the University of Cape Town. As a clinical psychologist, she develops and evaluates evidence-based psychosocial interventions for chronic illness and mental health, with a focus on marginalised communities. Her work primarily spans sub-Saharan Africa and includes a focus on supporting care in humanitarian settings.

Tea Chikviladze is a medical doctor and health expert with over ten years of clinical experience more than 15 years of experience in humanitarian health programming. Since 2008, Dr Chikviladze has managed and coordinated Community Health and First Aid activities at the Georgia Red Cross Society and actively participated in different humanitarian response operations across the country.

Tania Aase Dræbel is a sociologist employed as Assistant Professor at the University of Copenhagen. Her research explores access to health from a qualitative perspective, focusing on the relations, structures, and processes that shape it.

Bishal Gyawali is a leading expert in global health and implementation science, with a robust research portfolio focused on community-based management of non-communicable diseases among vulnerable and forcibly displaced populations. His work integrates participatory approaches to develop and implement context-specific models of care, addressing social determinants of health and health disparities. Dr Gyawali is deeply committed to developing equitable and sustainable solutions for chronic disease care in low-resource settings.

Johanna Hanefeld is a health policy analyst, and some of her research has focused on migration and health systems. She is an honorary Professor of Global Health Policy at the London School of Hygiene and Tropical Medicine. She is also Head of the Centre for International Health Protection at the Robert Koch-Institute in Berlin and is acting Vice-President.

Saria Hassan is Assistant Professor at the Emory School of Medicine and Rollins School of Public Health. She is a physician and an implementation science researcher whose work focuses on addressing the needs of persons living with non-communicable diseases in the setting of, and displaced by, climate-related disasters. Dr Hassan received her Medical Degree from Harvard Medical School and Master of Public Health from the London School of Tropical Medicine and Hygiene.

Ye Htut Oo is a dedicated public health researcher with experience in substance abuse prevention and control, mental health, and non-communicable diseases. He is a candidate for a doctorate in public health (DrPH) and holds masters degrees in Public Health (Global Health) and Rural Development Management. He has a particular interest in improving mental health services for underserved and socially marginalised groups. He has managed mental health projects for drug-affected communities and refugees with non-communicable diseases in Myanmar and Thailand.

David Kyaddondo has more than 20 years of experience in university teaching, research, and development social work. His research interests are in the areas of community linkages with health systems, HIV/AIDS, youth and children, disability, and technology. Most of his research projects involve collaborations with different universities and institutions, from both the north and the south. He holds a masters in medical anthropology, a PhD in anthropology, and was a postdoc fellow at the Wissenschaftskolleg in Berlin.

Usama Lubbad is a paediatric and child nutrition specialist and researcher with over 20 years of experience at UNRWA, Gaza. He has held leadership roles, contributed to international research, and published studies on diabetes and child health. Dr Lubbad holds professional diplomas in Family Medicine and Child health and Nutrition and actively participates in global medical conferences.

Davron Mukhamadiev is a health expert with more than 30 years of experience within the International Red Cross Red Crescent Movement. He has coordinated Red Cross Red Crescent Health operations across the Europe Region and held various roles in humanitarian response actions in Tajikistan, Sudan, Russian Federation, Belarus, and the South Caucasus. His expertise includes health in emergencies, mental health, and the psychosocial rehabilitation of vulnerable populations. Davron Mukhamadiev holds a Doctor of Medical Science degree and is the author of four books and more than 140 scientific articles in different scientific magazines.

Rita Nakanjako is an anthropologist and Lecturer in the Department of Sociology and Anthropology, Makerere University Kampala, Uganda. She has particular interest is empowerment of women and girls, the health-seeking behaviour of child migrants, the mental health of young people, chronic disease care among forcibly displaced populations, as well as cross-border studies. She has vast experience in conducting research among refugee and host communities in Uganda.

Esther Kalule Nanfuka is a professional social worker and Lecturer in the Department of Social Work and Social Administration, Makerere University in Kampala Uganda. Her areas of interest include resilience, social protection – particularly child and youth protection, gender-based violence, mental health of adolescents and young people, social health including HIV/AIDS, and other chronic diseases. She has been actively involved in conducting research among refugees and host communities of Uganda.

Jacqueline Ntombizodwa Ndlovu is a global health researcher with experience in scaling mental health and psychosocial support interventions through multi-sectoral integration. She works to strengthen the social dimensions of health responses in humanitarian crisis settings, with a particular interest in ensuring continuity of support across humanitarian and health systems.

Marie Louise Nørredam is a medical doctor and Professor at the University of Copenhagen. Her interests lie within the field of equity and health, migration and health, and health services research. She has a particular focus on the impact of ethnicity and migration on health conditions and access to health care, as well as vulnerable migrant groups, and their mental health and chronic disease risks.

Emmanuel Raju is a social scientist working to untangle the drivers of disasters. Emmanuel is currently the Director of the Copenhagen Centre for Disaster Research (COPE) at the University of Copenhagen. He works on issues of disaster risk creation and reduction, vulnerability and politics of disasters; and is interested in issues of integration of climate change adaptation and disaster risk reduction. He has conducted research in South Asia and East and Southern Africa.

Dricile Ratib is a public health researcher and Senior Lecturer at Muni University in Uganda, where he also serves as Acting Dean of the Faculty of Health Science. His work focuses on nutrition and the integration of interventions for communicable and non-communicable diseases, particularly in underserved and rural communities.

Santino Severoni is Director of the Department of Health and Migration at the World Health Organization in Geneva. He is a medical doctor and experienced system manager with over 25 years of experience as an international senior technical advisor and executive, having worked for governments, multilateral organisations, nongovernmental organisations, and foundations in Africa, the Balkans, Central Asia, and Europe.

Morten Skovdal is a community health psychologist and Professor of Participatory Health Research at the University of Copenhagen. He has a particular interest in involving underserved and socially marginalised groups in research, both to challenge dominant narratives and to attune interventions to their lived realities.

Nana Tsanava is a medical doctor and health expert with more than 30 years of experience in clinical care and humanitarian health programmes. She has worked with the International Red Cross Red Crescent Movement, Doctors Without Borders, and Project HOPE. She has coordinated and managed the health programmes in Europe, Central Asia, Asia-Pacific, South Caucasus, Middle East, Russian Federation, and Ukraine. Her primary focus areas are on community health and health in emergencies.

Susan Reynolds Whyte is Professor at the Department of Anthropology at the University of Copenhagen and conducts research in Uganda on social efforts to secure well-being in the face of poverty, disease, conflict, forced displacement, and rapid change. Her publications deal with the management of misfortune, legacies of violence, healthcare, and transformations in relations of gender and generation. She has worked on collaborative projects with Ugandan universities for 25 years.

Acknowledgements

This edited book builds on the symposium Continuity of Chronic Health Care among forcibly displaced populations, which was held in Copenhagen on 14 September 2023. We are deeply grateful to all the symposium participants for their insightful contributions, engaging discussions, and the collegial spirit that made the event so enriching. Special thanks go to Morten Mechlenborg Nørulf and the School of Global Health team for their invaluable assistance in planning and coordinating the symposium. We also extend our sincere appreciation to the Novo Nordisk Foundation (grant number NNF22OC0081196), whose generous support made both the symposium and the open-access publication of this book possible. Their commitment to fostering knowledge sharing and equity in healthcare has been instrumental in bringing this project to fruition. Finally, we would like to acknowledge the use of the following generative AI applications for writing and language support: Grammarly, an add-in application for writing assistance (grammar, syntax); and ChatGPT or Copilot, to rephrase specific paragraphs more concisely.

Foreword

Santino Severoni

In a time of unprecedented global displacement – where over 120 million people are forcibly uprooted due to conflict, persecution, environmental crises, and economic instability – the health of refugees and displaced populations stands as both a human rights priority and a public health necessity. Among the most urgent and complex challenges is the continuity of care for individuals living with chronic diseases, whose health trajectories are often severely disrupted by forced migration.

This edited volume, *Continuity of Care for Forcibly Displaced Persons Living with Chronic Illness*, offers an evidence-based and practice-informed response to that challenge. Through rigorous empirical studies and insightful case examples, the book underscores a core message that resonates deeply with the World Health Organization's (WHO) global work on health and migration: chronic care for displaced populations is not a peripheral concern – it is central to the integrity, inclusiveness, and resilience of health systems worldwide.

At the WHO, we have long advocated for the integration of migrants and forcibly displaced populations into national health systems, not only as a rights-based obligation but as a strategy to strengthen health security and universal health coverage (UHC). Our *Global Research Agenda on Health and Migration*, shaped in consultation with Member States, lays out a bold vision: that health responses to displacement must be holistic, coordinated across sectors, informed by data, and embedded in systems that can guarantee continuity, equity, and dignity.

The research compiled in this volume brings that vision to life. By applying social practice theory, the authors offer a novel lens through which to understand engagement with chronic disease care – as a dynamic and situated process shaped by personal agency, social relationships, and institutional configurations. These findings align with WHO's own review of country practices, as reflected in our *Global Evidence Review on Health and Migration* dashboard, which documents a growing number of national policies aimed at inclusive service delivery.

Indeed, there is a positive shift underway. As the WHO global dashboard illustrates, countries across all regions – such as Colombia, Portugal, Thailand, Uganda, and Türkiye – are advancing reforms to include refugees and other displaced populations in their national health plans, insurance schemes, and chronic disease programmes. This trend reflects an emerging consensus: that continuity of care for displaced populations is not only feasible, but beneficial to health systems at large. These inclusive practices strengthen preparedness, promote social cohesion, and reduce long-term costs by preventing disease progression and complications.

The chapters in this book are not merely academic exercises – they are actionable insights. Whether through the role of community health workers in Uganda, the integration of mental health in refugee care, or the structural innovations led by the Red Cross in Georgia, each chapter offers a concrete pathway toward equitable and sustained chronic disease care.

As we work collectively to implement the Global Action Plan on promoting the health of refugees and migrants, this volume serves as both a knowledge resource and a call to action. It reminds us that continuity of care for the displaced is not the responsibility of any single actor – it is a shared obligation that demands systems thinking, inclusive governance, and persistent advocacy.

I commend the editors and contributors for their dedication to evidence, equity, and innovation. By centring the lived realities of forcibly displaced persons, this book brings us closer to health systems that are truly for all – especially those too often left behind.

ONE

Working holistically: dimensions shaping continuity of care for forcibly displaced persons living with chronic illness

Morten Skovdal, Saria Hassan, Johanna Hanefeld, and
Lena Skovgaard Andersen

Forcibly displaced persons living with chronic illness face numerous challenges in maintaining continuity of care. This edited volume focuses on one of the most critical: their engagement with health services along the migratory journey. We approach engagement with health services as a social practice, showing how navigational capacities, social relations, and programmatic organisation shape whether and how such engagement becomes both desirable and possible. The chapters further demonstrate how the socio-cultural, political, economic, and policy landscapes of particular contexts condition these dynamics. Each contribution is structured around a form of 'work' or strategy that the authors identify as central to sustaining care continuity. Collectively, the chapters highlight the multiple dimensions that enable continuity of care, offering policy makers and practitioners a vocabulary for action.

Introduction

The global crisis of forced displacement has reached an alarming scale, with an estimated 122.6 million individuals uprooted from their homes due to war, conflict, economic crises, and climate-related disasters. This figure has nearly doubled in the past decade (UNHCR, 2025). Such displacement poses a severe threat to the health and well-being of those affected, as the migratory process increases the risk of non-communicable and infectious diseases and disrupts continuity of care and medication access for those with pre-existing chronic conditions (Zimmerman et al, 2011; Cantor et al, 2021).

Forcibly displaced persons experience fragmented and inconsistent access to healthcare across the full migratory journey – from displacement and transit, through resettlement, and into possible onward movement such as return or circular migration (Chiarenza et al, 2019). Despite ongoing and worsening challenges, our understanding of how to maintain consistent access to quality care for displaced persons with chronic diseases remains limited. Against this background, we, together with the School of Global Health at the University of Copenhagen, convened a symposium on 14 September 2023, with support from the Novo Nordisk Foundation. The symposium brought together leading experts, interdisciplinary researchers, and practitioners to present and reflect on the current state of research, policy, and practice in chronic disease care for forcibly displaced populations. The symposium comprised two keynote presentations, ten carefully selected presentations, and 12 poster presentations.[1] This edited book brings together some of the research presented at the symposium. The chapters are diverse. Five chapters report on new empirical research, two provide practitioner perspectives, and one chapter reviews existing literature. Broadly speaking, the chapters address three major health areas: diabetes, HIV, and mental health. This is no coincidence, as they reflect the pressing knowledge gaps, displacement patterns, and disease burdens of our time. Russia's invasion of Ukraine – a country heavily affected by HIV – has disrupted access to essential HIV treatment and prevention. In response, many neighbouring and European countries have had to ensure treatment access for displaced Ukrainians living with HIV (UNAIDS, 2025). The rise in armed conflicts and forced displacement has also contributed to growing levels of emotional distress, underscoring the urgent need for mental health services that are responsive to the diverse backgrounds and experiences of displaced populations. Diabetes presents another critical challenge, with prevalence rising and treatment gaps are widening, especially in low- and middle-income countries where the majority of displaced people are found. A recent global analysis of diabetes trends reports a fourfold increase in the number of adults living with the disease since 1990 (Zhou et al, 2024).

The chapters demonstrate that, despite the recognition of the importance of access to high-quality health services to manage HIV, mental distress, or diabetes, very often, displaced populations do not have equal and unfettered access to these services. We turn to social practice theory to unpack the interconnected nature of factors determining displaced populations' varied engagement with health services for the continuity of chronic disease care. There is no unified theory of practice (Shove, Pantzar, and Watson, 2012), but a broad consensus that practice theory draws attention to the background elements, or dimensions, that condition and shape behaviour (Nicolini, 2012; Blue et al, 2016; Skovdal, 2019), such as the practice of engaging with health services. The chapters of the book identify navigational capacities, social relations, and programmatic organisation as three key dimensions, or spheres of influence, that determine the degree to which displaced populations maintain or join the practice of engaging with health services. We summarise the main findings from these chapters according to these three dimensions to illustrate their role in explaining the importance and the potential pathways to establishing engagement with health services for forcibly displaced persons. As reflected in the chapter titles, each chapter speaks to a specific type of work the authors have identified as a key enabler of these spheres of influence.

Spheres of influence shaping engagement with health services for chronic disease care

Navigational capacities

Chapters One and Two highlight that forcibly displaced persons, as individuals, have different experiences and levels of health literacy, which shape their navigational capacities, motivations, and beliefs regarding engagement with health services for chronic disease care. These considerations can be crucial in defining strategies to enhance individuals' capacities to navigate and engage with health services successfully. Lubbard (Chapter Two) describes how socio-cultural, religious, and lifestyle factors negatively affect patients' beliefs and attitudes towards diabetes management, which in turn undermines their agentic capability to engage with their diabetes care. To turn this around, Lubbard provides details of a patient education and counselling intervention designed to improve the agentic capability of patients to adhere to their treatment. Lubbard finds that by addressing common misconceptions about diabetes treatment and fostering a deeper understanding of medication, lifestyle changes, and the prevention of complications, it is possible to strengthen the capacity for diabetes patients to engage with their treatment, improving adherence levels and treatment outcomes.

While the displaced people living with diabetes in Gaza demonstrated low levels of health literacy, the opposite is true for some of the displaced Ukrainians in Anderberg's chapter. In Chapter Three, Anderberg and colleagues explore how Ukrainians living with HIV manage to maintain continuity of

HIV care after being displaced from Ukraine following Russia's invasion in 2022. Through interviews with Ukrainians now living in Denmark, they find that the motivation to survive and remain on treatment is a strong guiding force for their agentic capability to navigate complex healthcare systems. Before fleeing Ukraine, they planned in meticulous detail, securing additional supplies of antiretroviral treatment. If they ran out of medication during transit, they actively contacted health services, notably the Red Cross, requesting access to treatment. Upon their arrival in Denmark, they skilfully navigated the healthcare system to their advantage, despite it being alien to them. Anderberg et al (Chapter Three) note qualitatively that Ukrainian refugees who have lived with HIV for a while, and have experienced the benefits of HIV care continuity, are motivated to sustain continuity of care and have the necessary experience to navigate access to HIV treatment before, during and after their flight. They call for greater recognition of, and attention to, the role of motivation and agency in shaping engagement with chronic disease care services.

The chapters by Lubbard and Anderberg et al demonstrate how health literacy, including an understanding of how treatment affects health outcomes, influences the motivation and capacity of displaced populations to navigate, act intentionally, and effectively access health services. Moreover, they emphasise that health literacy on its own is not enough to ensure access to care, but that characteristics such as agency and perseverance are also necessary. Both chapters draw attention to the knowledge, beliefs, and attitudes of individuals and how they shape an individual's engagement with health services for care continuity. However, individuals do not operate in a vacuum but are inextricably dependent on the availability of health services and support.

Social relations

Chapters Four and Five highlight how engagement with chronic disease care services for forcibly displaced populations is an inherently social and relational practice that can be promoted through community health workers (CHWs). In exploring the role of CHWs in ensuring continuity of care for refugees living with hypertension and diabetes in the Bidibidi refugee settlement in Uganda, Dræbel et al (Chapter Four) find that CHWs perform three critical roles. First, CHWs perform what the authors term relational work; they develop deep connections with local communities and build bridges between patients and healthcare workers. They provide encouragement, facilitate communication between healthcare workers and patients, and advocate for patients in their roles as intermediaries. The authors also find that CHWs perform critical chronic disease management functions, such as monitoring adherence, delivering medication, and referring complex cases. Finally, CHWs support health promotion activities at the community level by facilitating adherence to a healthy lifestyle. Dræbel et al find that formal health service delivery in Bidibidi and the health of patients living there rely heavily on this critical community work, done by a cadre of CHWs who receive little support and recognition for their central role.

While CHWs play a critical role in ensuring that patients stay engaged with a clinic and with their treatment, interpreters within the clinic also help forge a relationship between healthcare providers and patients. This is the topic of investigation in the chapter by Nakanjako et al (Chapter Five). Also drawing on research with refugees in Uganda, Nakanjako et al examine opportunities and challenges for interpreters to support patient-provider communication that enables continuity of care. The authors find that interpreters play a critical but difficult role in mediating patient-provider communication. They are refugees themselves, live in the local community, but are employed by the Ugandan health services. These different roles and identities affect how providers and patients experience and trust the interpretation. Refugee patients believe the interpreters, because of their shared language and culture, are 'one of them' and should be ready to advocate for their interests, but do not find this to be the case. Sometimes the relationship was perceived to be too close, making it difficult for some patients to speak freely in the presence of interpreters. Nakanjako et al call for more resources and greater attention to the critical role of interpreters in mediating patient-provider communication and relationships, as they are central to patients' continuity of care.

Programmatic organisation for patient-centred care

Chapters Four and Five report on research conducted in Uganda, a country at the forefront of health service provision for refugees with the highest concentration of refugees in Africa (WHO, 2024). However, access to chronic disease care services and treatment is not a given in all humanitarian settings. The chapter by Mukhamadiev and colleagues (Chapter Six) provides a practitioner perspective on how the Red Cross in Georgia has responded to undocumented Ukrainian refugees living with HIV, for whom the absence of legal status as refugees compromised their continuity of HIV care. The chapter presents a case study of how an external actor can facilitate and support processes that promote continuity of care. The Red Cross had to navigate significant challenges in Georgia due to the denial of health services for undocumented refugees (including Ukrainians), including HIV services, combined with widespread HIV stigma and health information barriers. This required the Red Cross to establish close and supportive relationships with local communities and authorities. Mukhamadiev et al describe the specific activities and costs involved with the delivery of HIV services by the Red Cross to ensure continuity of HIV care for displaced Ukrainians. However, the authors recognise that their efforts are unsustainable and call for policy change and long-term solutions that make it possible for all displaced individuals, regardless of their legal status, to access HIV services through national health programmes.

One of the services offered by the Red Cross in Georgia was psychosocial support, given the critical impact of mental health on the continuity of HIV care. This recognition of the deep interconnections between physical and psychological health is also covered by Htut Oo (Chapter Seven). Htut Oo, in a review of literature and guidelines, argues that providers of post-migration chronic disease care services, across the spectrum of prevention, treatment, and rehabilitation, *must* address mental health as a critical factor affecting continuity of care for refugees with chronic conditions. She goes on to argue that chronic disease care for forcibly displaced persons must be integrated with mental health and psychosocial support (MHPSS) services. She further justifies this approach of programmatic integration by discussing how it adheres to principles of community-led and person-centred chronic disease care that underpin successful health outcomes.

While Htut Oo recognises the role of addressing mental health to improve access to care for other chronic health conditions, Ndlovu (Chapter Eight) addresses the high prevalence of psychological distress requiring attention among displaced persons. Ndlovu presents a case study of how multi-sectoral integration can support continued engagement with MHPSS services. Drawing on research of a guided self-help intervention (SH+) for refugees in Uganda, Ndlovu examines some of the pathways through which integrating a mental health intervention into an economic and livelihoods project, as well as a social protection project, can achieve continuity of mental health care. She argues that integrating MHPSS services into broader resilience-building initiatives such as economic empowerment, social support, and education makes mental health services more accessible and relevant, and less stigmatised, ultimately enhancing engagement and continuity of mental health care.

Working holistically for continuity of care

Reporting on findings and reflections from different humanitarian and chronic disease contexts, this collection of chapters has identified various strategies, framed as types of work, that shape the ability of forcibly displaced persons to maintain continuity of care for chronic diseases during transit or in host communities. Rather than approaching care continuity as solely the responsibility or trait of individuals, for instance through disease self-management, the chapters note three requisite dimensions that structure opportunities for care continuity: the agency of patients, relationality and community structures, and programmatic organisation to deliver patient-centred care (see Figure 1.1).

Although each chapter makes a case for a strategy based on a specific humanitarian and chronic disease context, our extrapolation of requisite dimensions encourages us, with the help of social practice theory, to argue that understanding how care continuity through engagement with chronic disease care services takes hold is a matter of understanding how different strategies, covering all three dimensions, are available and coordinated. For instance, without access to essential medicines, care from a biomedical treatment perspective comes to a halt. Equally, medicines may be available, but if patients' mental health is compromised and they cannot find the motivation to go to the clinic, the work done to ensure access to essential medicines is undermined. Determining the types of work required to support the continuity of care for forcibly displaced persons in a given context involves understanding how different strategies across the three requisite dimensions interconnect and influence each other. Only by addressing the interplay between these dimensions can we develop sustainable patient-centred and context-sensitive models of care that meet the needs of forcibly displaced persons living with chronic disease. This inevitably necessitates a holistic response, requiring actors from different sectors to collaborate and coordinate, as evidenced throughout the following chapters.

Figure 1.1: Spheres of influence and types of work for a holistic response to the continuity of care for forcibly displaced persons living with chronic illness

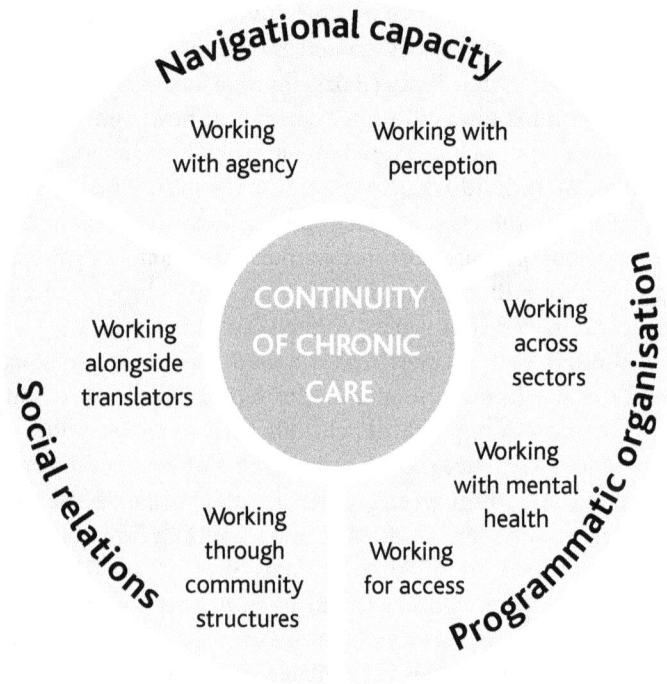

Note
1. See https://globalhealth.ku.dk/events/2023/ucph-global-health-day for more detail about the symposium.

References

Blue, S., Shove, E., Carmona, C., and Kelly, M. P. (2016). Theories of practice and public health: Understanding (un) healthy practices. *Critical Public Health*, 26(1), 36–50.

Cantor, D., Swartz, J., Roberts, B., Abbara, A., Ager, A., Bhutta, Z.A., ... Smith, J. (2021). Understanding the health needs of internally displaced persons: A scoping review. *Journal of Migration and Health*, 4, 100071. doi:10.1016/j.jmh.2021.100071

Chiarenza, A., Dauvrin, M., Chiesa, V., Baatout, S., and Verrept, H. (2019). Supporting access to healthcare for refugees and migrants in European countries under particular migratory pressure. *BMC Health Services Research*, *19*(1), 513. doi:10.1186/s12913-019-4353-1

Nicolini, D. (2012). *Practice theory, work, and organization: An introduction*. Oxford University Press.

Shove, E., Pantzar, M., and Watson, M. (2012). *The dynamics of social practice: Everyday life and how it changes*. Sage Publications.

Skovdal, M. (2019). Facilitating engagement with PrEP and other HIV prevention technologies through practice-based combination prevention. *Journal of the International AIDS Society*, *22*(S4), e25294. doi:10.1002/jia2.25294

UNAIDS (2025). *Ensuring the HIV response and healthcare stability: From crisis to prospective recovery*. UNAIDS.

UNHCR (2024). *Mid-Year Trends 2024*. UNHCR Global Data Service: Copenhagen.

WHO (2024). Refugee and migrant health system review: Challenges and opportunities for long-term health system strengthening in Uganda. World Health Organization.

Zhou, B., Rayner, A.W., Gregg, E.W., Sheffer, K.E., … Ezzati, M. (2024). Worldwide trends in diabetes prevalence and treatment from 1990 to 2022: A pooled analysis of 1108 population-representative studies with 141 million participants. *The Lancet*, *404*(10467), 2077–2093. doi:10.1016/S0140-6736(24)02317-1

Zimmerman, C., Kiss, L., and Hossain, M. (2011). Migration and health: A framework for 21st century policy-making. *PLoS Medicine*, *8*(5), e1001034.

PART I

Navigational capacity

TWO

Working with perceptions: patient education and counselling as pathways to continuity of care among diabetic patients in Gaza

Usama Lubbad

This chapter explores the impact of health literacy on treatment adherence among refugees in Gaza living with diabetes. It evaluates how diabetes education can improve disease management, focusing on knowledge, attitudes, and behaviour changes. The study included 362 diabetic patients, with the majority being classified as overweight or obese based on standard body mass index (BMI) categories. Baseline results showed that 83.7 per cent of the sample had uncontrolled diabetes, and 67.6 per cent exhibited suboptimal adherence to their medication regimen. The diabetes education and counselling intervention involved educational sessions, social media groups, and mental health counselling. Post-intervention, 28.3 per cent of participants showed improved HbA1c levels, with 13.7 per cent achieving controlled diabetes status. The findings suggest effective patient education and counselling can improve adherence and glycaemic control.

Introduction

Diabetes mellitus (DM) is a chronic metabolic disorder characterised by hyperglycaemia, resulting from impaired insulin production or action. Management of diabetes requires a multifaceted approach, incorporating medication, lifestyle changes, and continuous monitoring. The primary goal of diabetes management is to achieve optimal glycaemic control to prevent or delay complications such as neuropathy, nephropathy, cardiovascular disease, and retinopathy. Effective management not only reduces the risk of long-term complications but also improves patients' quality of life (Chantzaras and Yfantopoulos, 2022).

Although patient education has long been considered critical to the success of diabetes management, limited access to health education, resources, and services hinders effective diabetes management among refugees and displaced individuals in regions such as the Middle East and the Gaza Strip, in particular. As a result, there is a substantial discrepancy between the availability of medical treatment and the patients' capacity to achieve long-term glycaemic control. There is an urgent need to identify and evaluate effective health education initiatives for Palestinian refugees in the region.

Diabetes care is persistently neglected in humanitarian crises despite the growing prevalence of diabetes and the increasing number of displaced populations, particularly in low- and middle-income countries (Kehlenbrink et al, 2023). Kehlenbrink and colleagues identify four key factors contributing to this neglect: evolving paradigms in humanitarian health care, complexities in delivering diabetes services in crisis settings, social and cultural barriers, and inadequate financing. Humanitarian organisations lack standardised guidelines for diabetes care, leading to significant variability in service provision. Without intervention, people living with diabetes (PLWD) will continue to experience health inequities in crisis settings. The authors emphasise the need for contingency planning within health systems to ensure continuity of diabetes care during emergencies, integrating diabetes management into emergency preparedness plans at both national and international levels. By addressing these challenges, practical and feasible opportunities exist to improve diabetes care in humanitarian settings, reinforcing the humanitarian imperative that action must be taken to prevent avoidable suffering and uphold health equity for PLWD.

This chapter will explore how a diabetes education initiative at the SABRA healthcare centre, part of the United Nations Relief and Works Agency for Palestine Refugees in the Near East (UNRWA) in Gaza, helped reshape patients' perceptions of their disease and influenced their glycaemic control outcomes. By focusing on the link between education, medication adherence, and glycaemic control, the study highlights the importance of working with patients' perceptions of their treatment to manage chronic diseases effectively.

Medication adherence and glycaemic control in humanitarian settings

Medication adherence is critical in maintaining glycaemic control in patients with diabetes. Consistent use of prescribed medications, particularly insulin and oral hypoglycaemics, helps regulate blood glucose levels, reduce complications, and improve overall health outcomes. However, research shows that adherence to diabetes medications is often suboptimal among patients in humanitarian settings (Lyles et al, 2020). Since 2007, the Gaza Strip has been subject to significant movement and access restrictions, recurrent armed conflicts, and limited access to essential services, thus constituting a particular humanitarian setting that affects the quality and availability of health services for PLWD. Until the war broke out in 2023, the living conditions for Palestinians in Gaza were already dire and characterised by longstanding structural and economic challenges, including a severely constrained healthcare system. Presently, though not a focus of this chapter, Gaza has turned into a humanitarian disaster at an unprecedented scale.

The prevalence of chronic disease is on the rise, making it a significant concern in global health. For instance, between 1990 and 2022, the number of persons living with diabetes increased from 200 million to 830 million (WHO, 2024). Pharmacotherapy is a regular component of long-term treatment plans for many chronic diseases. Suboptimal adherence prevents many patients from realising the full therapeutic benefits of medications, even when these treatments are effective in managing chronic disease. Between 35 and 70 per cent of people with hypertension (HTN) and 36–93 per cent of those with type 2 diabetes mellitus (DMT2) have been reported to adhere adequately to their treatment plans (Mann et al, 2009; Hsiao et al, 2012). Half or more of chronic obstructive pulmonary disease patients do not take their medicine as prescribed, and many more do not know how to use their inhalers properly (Krauskopf et al, 2015). Similarly, non-adherence to asthma preventive medicine affects 30–70 per cent of patients (Feehan et al, 2015). Significant disease deterioration, treatment failure, more hospitalisations, and higher health care expenses are all outcomes of suboptimal adherence (Kardas et al, 2013).

Many facets influence medication adherence. Illness perceptions, health literacy, self-efficacy, cognitive abilities (including memory, coping, and problem-solving skills), and psychosocial variables (such as personal and cultural views related to medicine use) all play a role in medication adherence (Chia et al, 2006). Patients' subjective views about their health may influence their acceptance of medical recommendations, including the use of medications. A study by Lyles and colleagues (2020) analysed data from a 2015 household survey of Syrian refugees and Lebanese host communities. The study examined differences in care-seeking, health facility utilisation, out-of-pocket payments for care, and medication interruption. The results revealed significant disparities, with refugees facing more difficulties in accessing care and experiencing higher rates of medication interruption. While host community members had better access to care, they faced significantly higher out-of-pocket costs. Refugees primarily sought care at primary health facilities due to cost considerations, while host community members preferred private clinics for better quality and continuity of care. The study concludes that efforts should focus on reducing health service costs for refugees and vulnerable host community members, along with improving communication about available subsidised care (Lyles et al, 2020).

Before the current war, the SABRA healthcare centre in Gaza observed that a large proportion of diabetes patients exhibited poor medication adherence. Low adherence not only exacerbates uncontrolled glycemia but also contributes to a cycle of poor health outcomes and increased healthcare costs. Addressing the underlying causes of low adherence is critical to improving glycaemic control among diabetes patients.

In Gaza, where cultural, socio-economic, and psychological factors heavily influence healthcare behaviours, patients' beliefs about their medications and attitudes toward disease management are crucial to understanding adherence patterns. Many patients may not fully comprehend the importance of consistent medication use, while others may be influenced by misinformation or mistrust toward healthcare providers.

Importance of addressing beliefs and attitudes towards diabetes care

Beliefs and attitudes toward disease management are pivotal in determining how well patients adhere to medical recommendations. Cultural factors, religious beliefs, psychological barriers, and personal experiences shape a patient's perception of diabetes care. For instance, some individuals may believe that diabetes is a condition that cannot be managed effectively, while others may rely on traditional remedies instead of modern medical treatment (Al-Sahouri et al, 2019).

In the Middle Eastern context, where diabetes management is often influenced by cultural, religious, and lifestyle factors such as dietary restrictions and fasting, addressing these perceptions is crucial (Khdour et al, 2020; Alsaidan et al, 2023). By integrating culturally sensitive approaches into diabetes care, patients can be empowered to make informed decisions about their health. The diabetes education initiative, developed during the study period at SABRA healthcare centre, aimed to challenge these perceptions by offering accurate information about the condition and its management. Through strategies such as group discussions, one-on-one counselling, and mental health support, the programme aimed to enhance patients' knowledge and attitudes, ultimately leading to improved glycaemic outcomes.

Methodology

Study design and participant demographics

The study employed a quasi-experimental design with unmatched groups to evaluate an education and counselling intervention, targeting diabetes patients who regularly attended the SABRA healthcare centre under the UNRWA system in Gaza. The aim was to assess the impact of structured diabetes education and counselling on glycaemic control, with a specific focus on HbA1c levels before and after the intervention. The population included all age groups with both type 1 and type 2 diabetes.

The study's eligibility criteria were specifically designed to focus on diabetic patients aged 18 years and older, diagnosed with type 1 or type 2 diabetes, who had been attending the health centre for at least three months before the intervention. Participants were required to have been prescribed diabetes-related medications and treatments, including insulin, oral hypoglycaemics, and other diabetes-related therapeutic regimens. Patients with severe comorbidities, cognitive impairments, or those unable to attend the education sessions due to logistical or health issues were excluded from the study. Informed consent was obtained from all participants, and the UNRWA granted ethical approval.

Educational intervention strategies

The educational strategies employed in this intervention were designed to address the diverse needs of diabetes patients and the barriers they face in achieving glycaemic control. These strategies included:

- *Educational Sessions*: Regular group-based sessions were conducted to educate patients on the fundamentals of diabetes management, including understanding blood sugar levels, the role of insulin and oral medications, and the importance of a balanced diet and regular exercise. These sessions also provided an opportunity for patients to ask questions and share their experiences, fostering a sense of community and support.
- *Social Media Groups*: With limited access to in-person care due to infrastructure challenges in Gaza, social media platforms were utilised to create online support groups where patients could receive ongoing education, share their experiences, and stay connected with healthcare providers. These groups also facilitated the dissemination of educational materials in various formats, including videos, infographics, and written content.
- *Groups and One-on-One Meetings*: Group sessions were held to address common concerns and misconceptions about diabetes management. Additionally, one-on-one meetings with healthcare providers allowed for personalised education tailored to the specific needs of individual patients. This approach ensured that patients with complex health issues or unique barriers to care received the necessary attention.

- *Multidisciplinary Team Workshops*: Healthcare providers from various specialities, including endocrinologists, dietitians, psychologists, and nurses, collaborated in workshops designed to provide a holistic approach to diabetes management. These workshops emphasised the importance of teamwork in delivering comprehensive care and helped patients understand the different aspects of their treatment plans.

Procedure

The primary intervention involved a structured patient education programme, including counselling sessions and diabetes management workshops, aimed at enhancing patients' understanding of their condition, promoting medication adherence, and facilitating lifestyle modifications.

The intervention consisted of weekly educational sessions delivered by trained healthcare professionals, including doctors, nurses, and nutritionists, who provided individualised counselling. These sessions covered various topics, including the importance of medication adherence, dietary changes, exercise, and self-monitoring of blood glucose levels. Additionally, patients were provided with educational materials, including brochures and booklets, to reinforce the key points discussed during the sessions. The effectiveness of the intervention was evaluated using pre- and post-assessment surveys, patient interviews, and clinical data analysis, which focused on key metrics such as adherence to medication, blood glucose control, and health-related quality of life.

Data collection and analysis

Data collection was carried out from March to June 2023, both before and after the intervention, to assess changes in glycaemic control. Baseline HbA1c levels were obtained from the UNRWA e-health system before the start of the intervention, allowing for a comparison with post-intervention HbA1c levels. The HbA1c test is a critical marker for long-term glucose control, providing insight into a patient's average blood sugar levels over the past 2–3 months.

The study employed a convenience sampling method, recruiting patients who were willing to participate in the intervention and meet the eligibility criteria. The data collection tools included structured questionnaires to assess patients' knowledge, attitudes, and practices regarding diabetes management before and after the intervention. A control group of diabetic patients who did not receive the educational programme was also included for comparison to evaluate the impact of the intervention on the outcomes of interest. Data analysis was conducted using both qualitative and quantitative methods, including descriptive statistics and inferential tests to determine the significance of changes in medication adherence and glycaemic control among participants.

Data analysis was conducted using SPSS v23 software, ensuring rigorous statistical analysis of the intervention's outcomes. Frequency analyses were performed for sociodemographic characteristics as well as mean and standard deviations for continuous variables. Chi-square test was used to test for relationships, while independent t-test and one-way ANOVA were used to compare means.

Results

Baseline characteristics of participants

A total of 362 participants were included in the study, which initially invited 400 participants, with a median age of 50 years. The demographic distribution revealed that more than half of the participants were female (54.1 per cent). Furthermore, the BMI analysis, assessed by data collectors' measurements, showed that over two-thirds of the participants were classified as either overweight (38.1 per cent) or obese (37.8 per cent), both of which are known risk factors for poor glycaemic control. This sample was representative of the broader diabetes population in Gaza, where socio-economic challenges, limited access to healthcare, and high rates of obesity contribute to the growing burden of diabetes.

At baseline, most participants exhibited poor glycaemic control, with 83.7 per cent of the cohort having HbA1c levels greater than 7 per cent, indicative of uncontrolled diabetes. This baseline data underscores the pressing need for effective intervention strategies to help these patients manage their condition.

In terms of medication adherence, 67.6 per cent of participants were classified as having low adherence to their prescribed diabetes medications. Notably, none of the participants were found to have high adherence levels. These findings highlight the significant gap between treatment recommendations and patient behaviour, which likely contributed to the poor glycaemic control observed in the cohort.

Post-intervention improvements in HbA1c levels

Following the implementation of the educational interventions, there were notable improvements in the participants' glycemic control. Overall, 28.3 per cent of patients experienced a reduction in their HbA1c levels, with an average decrease from 8.2 per ccent to 7.3 per cent. While only 13.7 per cent of participants achieved the target HbA1c level of less than 7 per cent, an additional 14.6 per cent of participants showed improvement in their HbA1c levels, although they had not yet reached the controlled status.

These results suggest that while the educational intervention did not result in immediate glycemic control for all participants, it led to meaningful improvements in a substantial proportion of the cohort. Furthermore, the fact that no patients exhibited high adherence to their medications at baseline, but improvements were observed post-intervention, points to the efficacy of the education initiative in promoting better adherence and understanding of diabetes management.

A paired t-test was performed to compare the mean HbA1c levels before and after the intervention. The analysis revealed a statistically significant reduction in HbA1c levels among participants, with a mean decrease from 8.2 per cent pre-intervention to 7.3 per cent post-intervention ($p < 0.05$). This considerable reduction indicates the effectiveness of the diabetes education initiative in improving glycaemic control among the study population. Furthermore, an independent t-test was applied to assess differences in HbA1c improvement between male and female participants. The results showed no statistically significant difference ($p > 0.05$), suggesting that the intervention benefited both genders equally.

To examine the relationship between medication adherence and glycaemic control, a Chi-square test was conducted. The results indicated a significant association between improved adherence levels and better post-intervention glycaemic outcomes ($p < 0.05$). This finding highlights the crucial role of medication adherence in achieving glycaemic control and supports the importance of patient education and counselling in enhancing adherence behaviours.

Additionally, a one-way ANOVA was performed to determine whether there were significant differences in HbA1c improvement across different BMI categories. The analysis revealed a statistically significant difference among the groups ($p < 0.05$), indicating that patients with different BMI levels responded differently to the intervention. This suggests that obesity may influence glycaemic control responses, and tailored interventions may be necessary for overweight and obese patients.

Discussion

This study highlights the significant impact of educational interventions on diabetes management, particularly through addressing patients' beliefs and attitudes. Our findings demonstrate that structured educational strategies, including group sessions, one-on-one counselling, and mental health support, improved medication adherence and glycaemic control among patients in Gaza. By addressing common misconceptions about diabetes treatment and fostering a deeper understanding of medication, lifestyle changes, and the prevention of complications, the intervention improved HbA1c levels and overall health behaviours.

The positive relationship between patient education and improved glycaemic outcomes aligns with other studies in the region and among refugee populations. Previous research has also emphasised the importance of culturally tailored education in improving diabetes management in areas with limited healthcare access and high levels of displacement, such as the Gaza Strip. However, unlike studies focused solely on clinical education, our intervention included mental health support, which has proven essential in managing diabetes, as psychological factors like stress and anxiety can significantly affect medication adherence. This holistic approach distinguishes our findings from others and underscores the importance of addressing both physical and psychological barriers to care.

The success of this intervention highlights the importance of patient-centred care that addresses both the clinical and psychosocial aspects of chronic disease management. By integrating education with mental health support, healthcare providers can help patients navigate the complex demands of chronic disease management, particularly in low-resource settings. This model of care could be adapted for other conditions such as hypertension and cardiovascular disease, where medication adherence and lifestyle changes are similarly crucial.

The findings of this study underscore the substantial challenges associated with glycaemic control among diabetic patients at the SABRA healthcare centre, as well as the positive impact of targeted educational interventions on diabetes management. At baseline, a significant majority (83.7 per cent) of participants exhibited poor glycaemic control (HbA1c > 7%), indicating a considerable gap in effective diabetes self-management. Furthermore, the high prevalence of overweight (38.1 per cent) and obesity (37.8 per cent) within the study population reflects broader trends observed in diabetes patients, where excess weight is a known risk factor for insulin resistance and poor metabolic control. These findings align with existing literature emphasising the strong correlation between obesity and diabetes progression, particularly in resource-limited settings such as Gaza, where lifestyle factors and healthcare accessibility play a crucial role in disease outcomes.

A particularly concerning baseline finding was the low level of medication adherence, with 67.6 per cent of participants classified as having poor adherence and none exhibiting high adherence. Poor medication adherence has been well-documented as a significant barrier to achieving optimal glycaemic control, and these findings highlight the urgent need for interventions that improve patient engagement with their prescribed regimens. The significant association between medication adherence and glycaemic outcomes ($p < 0.05$) observed in this study further reinforces the importance of patient education and counselling in enhancing adherence behaviours. Interventions that address patients' beliefs about medications and their concerns about side effects, affordability, and trust in healthcare providers are critical for sustainable diabetes management.

The effectiveness of the educational initiative was demonstrated by the statistically significant reduction in mean HbA1c levels from 8.2 per cent pre-intervention to 7.3 per cent post-intervention ($p < 0.05$). Although only 13.7 per cent of participants achieved the target HbA1c level of <7 per cent, an additional 14.6 per cent exhibited meaningful improvements, suggesting that educational interventions can catalyse long-term diabetes management. The significant impact of the intervention on glycaemic control is consistent with prior studies showing that structured diabetes education programs enhance patients' knowledge, self-efficacy, and adherence to treatment recommendations (Baradaran et al, 2010).

Notably, no statistically significant differences were found between male and female participants regarding HbA1c improvement ($p > 0.05$), suggesting that the intervention was equally beneficial across genders. However, the results of the one-way ANOVA indicate that BMI had a significant effect on glycaemic control outcomes ($p < 0.05$), suggesting that overweight and obese individuals may require more intensive or personalised interventions to achieve similar improvements. Given the strong link between obesity and insulin resistance, future interventions should incorporate weight management strategies, including dietary counselling and physical activity promotion, to optimise diabetes care.

In the Gaza Strip, where limited healthcare access and economic hardship present ongoing challenges, tailoring education to the cultural and socio-economic needs of patients is essential. Remote education, such as social media groups and community-based sessions, proved effective in overcoming barriers to face-to-face care, especially in conflict settings. This approach emphasises the importance of continuous patient education, ensuring that patients remain engaged in managing their health.

This study demonstrates that targeted educational interventions can significantly improve glycaemic control among diabetes patients in resource-limited settings. Patients who participated in the initiative at SABRA healthcare centre exhibited marked improvements in HbA1c levels, which reflect better adherence to treatment plans and lifestyle modifications. The findings highlight the importance of addressing clinical and psychosocial barriers to effective diabetes management, such as economic constraints, cultural misconceptions, and mental health challenges.

The observed improvements align with prior research emphasising the efficacy of patient education in chronic disease management. For instance, studies conducted in refugee settings have shown that community-based education programmes can improve health outcomes despite limited resources. However, unlike similar interventions in other Middle Eastern contexts, this study integrated mental health support as a core component, addressing psychological barriers alongside clinical education.

Integrating mental health support into diabetes education underscores the need for continuity of care in resource-constrained and conflict-affected regions. This model ensures that patients receive not only one-time interventions, but also ongoing support tailored to their evolving needs. Continuity of care is particularly critical for displaced populations, as disruptions in care often exacerbate chronic disease progression in such settings. Future initiatives should prioritise sustainable education models, such as telehealth and community health worker programmes, to bridge gaps in access to care.

The Gaza Strip, home to over two million Palestinians, is a unique humanitarian context characterised by decades of displacement, conflict, and socio-economic challenges. Although Palestinians in Gaza have not crossed international borders, they are refugees under UNRWA mandate, having been displaced since 1948. This protracted refugee situation, compounded by a 16-year-long blockade and recurring escalations of violence, has severely impacted the population's ability to rebuild their lives and access basic services, including healthcare. These circumstances have created a humanitarian crisis where healthcare systems are overburdened, and chronic disease management, such as diabetes care, faces significant challenges.

The diabetes education initiative implemented at SABRA healthcare centre was specifically designed to address the unique needs of Palestinian refugees in this protracted crisis. The programme incorporated culturally tailored education acknowledging the community's history, language, and socio-economic struggles. For example, educational sessions were delivered in Arabic and referenced cultural and religious practices, such as fasting during Ramadan, to ensure relevance and resonance with participants. Moreover, including social media-based support groups provided a practical solution to the challenges of limited mobility and restricted access to in-person care in Gaza. This adaptation demonstrates that interventions designed with an understanding of the local humanitarian context can effectively address barriers to chronic disease management.

The findings of this study, while applicable to other resource-limited settings, are particularly significant in the context of refugees and displaced populations. Unlike many other refugee groups who cross borders, Palestinians in Gaza face unique constraints as an internally displaced population living under siege. The intervention's success in improving glycaemic control underscores the importance of designing health initiatives that integrate cultural sensitivity with practical solutions tailored to such contexts. This approach can inform diabetes management strategies for Palestinian refugees across the Middle East, where similar cultural, linguistic, and socio-economic conditions prevail.

This study adds to the growing literature on managing chronic diseases among refugees and in humanitarian settings. While existing research often focuses on acute healthcare needs in displacement contexts, this chapter emphasises the long-term challenges of chronic disease management. By addressing both the psychosocial and clinical aspects of care, the intervention aligns with studies highlighting the necessity of holistic, patient-centred approaches in refugee healthcare (Iqbal et al, 2022). However, it also advances the field by demonstrating the feasibility of integrating mental health support into diabetes education, a component often overlooked in similar interventions.

Study strengths and limitations

This study has several strengths, including its focus on both physical and psychological factors that affect diabetes management. However, a limitation is the lack of data specifically linking improvements in mental health to the educational intervention. While the inclusion of mental health support was a key aspect of the programme, we did not collect sufficient data to directly measure changes in psychological outcomes, which makes any claims regarding mental health improvement speculative. Future studies could benefit from incorporating specific mental health assessments to gain a deeper understanding of this relationship.

Future research should focus on assessing the long-term effects of educational interventions on both physical and psychological outcomes. Additionally, investigating the role of healthcare providers in fostering stronger patient-provider relationships could offer deeper, improved insights into how trust and communication influence treatment adherence. Expanding this model to other chronic diseases in refugee and conflict settings would be valuable, particularly in areas with limited healthcare infrastructure. It is recommended that healthcare systems prioritise comprehensive education programmes that integrate mental health support and offer ongoing follow-up care to enhance chronic disease management.

Challenges experienced and recommendations for future interventions

While the diabetes education initiative at SABRA healthcare centre demonstrated significant success in improving glycaemic control among patients, several challenges and limitations were noted that are worth addressing in future interventions.

- *Limited Resources and Accessibility*: In resource-limited settings, such as Gaza, access to healthcare services, medications, and educational materials can be challenging due to economic constraints, conflict, and infrastructure limitations. Although the education initiative utilised social media and remote communication tools, some patients may still have faced barriers in accessing these resources regularly.

Addressing these gaps will require innovative solutions, such as community-based outreach programmes or mobile health clinics, to ensure that all patients, regardless of their socio-economic status, receive the necessary support.

- *Cultural and Social Barriers*: Cultural beliefs and social stigmas surrounding diabetes may hinder some patients' ability to fully engage in education programmes or adhere to their treatment regimen. For example, some patients may hold traditional beliefs about illness and healing that conflict with modern medical recommendations. In such cases, healthcare providers must collaborate closely with community leaders and religious figures to develop culturally sensitive education programmes that resonate with patients and respect their beliefs.
- *Sustainability of the Intervention*: A key challenge for any educational initiative is ensuring its long-term sustainability. While the intervention at SABRA healthcare centre achieved notable short-term improvements in glycaemic control, maintaining these gains requires ongoing support and follow-up. Future programmes should focus on building local capacity and training healthcare providers to continue delivering education and support to patients beyond the initial intervention.
- *Patient Engagement and Motivation*: Despite the educational intervention's success, some patients may continue to struggle with motivation and adherence to diabetes management practices. Factors such as psychological distress, family responsibilities, and social pressures can impact a patient's ability to prioritise their health. Future initiatives should explore strategies to enhance patient motivation, such as peer support groups, incentive-based programmes, and personalised goal setting.

The diabetes education initiative at SABRA healthcare centre demonstrates the importance of integrating education, mental health support, and continuous follow-up in managing chronic diseases. By addressing the physical and psychological aspects of diabetes care, healthcare providers can help patients improve medication adherence, glycaemic control, and overall health outcomes. This approach has the potential to be adapted for use in other chronic conditions and healthcare settings, particularly in resource-limited regions where patient education can significantly impact disease management.

Conclusion

This study underscores the importance of addressing patient perceptions in diabetes management through targeted, structured education. The diabetes education initiative at SABRA healthcare centre in Gaza resulted in improvements, with 28.3 per cent of participants exhibiting better HbA1c levels and 13.7 per cent achieving controlled HbA1c status. These outcomes were achieved through a holistic approach combining educational sessions, social media engagement, one-on-one counselling, and mental health support. By reshaping patients' beliefs, enhancing their understanding of diabetes, and addressing psychological and social factors, the initiative empowered patients to take active control of their health, leading to improved adherence and glycaemic outcomes

Recommendations for future education initiatives

The study findings point to several recommendations for future education initiatives aimed at improving glycaemic control:

- *Culturally tailored education*: Educational programmes should be designed to meet the specific cultural, social, and economic needs of the patient population. For example, in Gaza, integrating religious and cultural beliefs about health into educational sessions can help bridge the gap between traditional practices and modern medical recommendations.

- *Multidisciplinary approach*: Effective chronic disease management requires collaboration across multiple healthcare disciplines. In future initiatives, healthcare providers should collaborate to offer a comprehensive education programme that encompasses not only medical information but also dietary guidance, physical activity recommendations, and mental health support.
- *Use of technology*: In areas where access to healthcare services is limited, technology plays a crucial role in patient education. The use of social media, telemedicine, and online support groups can help maintain continuous engagement with patients and provide them with the necessary resources to manage their condition.
- *Continuous follow-up and support*: Education should not be a one-time intervention but an ongoing process. Regular follow-ups, either in person or through digital platforms, can help reinforce the education provided, address new challenges, and ensure that patients remain engaged in their self-management.
- *Integration of mental health services*: Mental health counselling should be a core component of chronic disease management programmes. Addressing psychological barriers such as stress, anxiety, and depression can improve medication adherence, lifestyle modification, and overall health outcomes.
- *Exploring the role of family and caregivers*: Diabetes management often requires the support of family members or caregivers, particularly for patients who struggle to manage their condition independently. Future research could examine the role of family involvement in diabetes education and explore strategies for integrating caregivers into educational initiatives.
- *Technological innovations in education*: Technology, such as mobile apps, telemedicine, and wearable devices, holds great potential for enhancing patient education and monitoring in diabetes care. Future studies could explore how these technologies can be integrated into educational programmes

to provide real-time feedback and support for patients as they manage their condition.

- *Mental health and chronic disease management*: The integration of mental health counselling into the diabetes education initiative at the SABRA healthcare centre was a key factor in the intervention's success. Future research could further explore the intersection of mental health and chronic disease management, examining how addressing psychological distress and improving emotional well-being can enhance patient outcomes in diabetes and other chronic conditions.

References

Al-Sahouri, A., Merrell, J., and Snelgrove, S. (2019). Barriers to good glycemic control levels and adherence to diabetes management plan in adults with Type-2 diabetes in Jordan: A literature review. *Patient Preference and Adherence*, *13*, 675–693. https://doi.org/10.2147/PPA.S198828

Alsaidan, A.A., Alotaibi, S.F., Thirunavukkarasu, A., ALruwaili, B.F., … Alwushayh, Y.A. (2023). Medication adherence and its associated factors among patients with type 2 diabetes mellitus attending primary health centers of eastern province, Saudi Arabia. *Medicina*, *59*(5), 989.

Baradaran, H.R., Shams-Hosseini, N., Noori-Hekmat, S., Tehrani-Banihashemi, A., and Khamseh, M.E. (2010). Effectiveness of diabetes educational interventions in Iran: A systematic review. *Diabetes Technology & Therapeutics*, *12*(4), 317–331.

Chantzaras, A. and Yfantopoulos, J. (2022). Association between medication adherence and health-related quality of life of patients with diabetes. *Hormones*, *21*(4), 691–705.

Chia, L., Schlenk, E.A., and Dunbar-Jacob, J. (2006). Effect of personal and cultural beliefs on medication adherence in the elderly. *Drugs & Aging*, *23*, 191–202.

Feehan, M., Ranker, L., Durante, R., Cooper, D., Jones, G., Young, D., and Munger, M. (2015). Adherence to controller asthma medications: 6-month prevalence across a US community pharmacy chain. *Journal of Clinical Pharmacy and Therapeutics*, *40*(5), 590–593.

Hsiao, C.-Y., Chang, C., and Chen, C.-D. (2012). An investigation on illness perception and adherence among hypertensive patients. *The Kaohsiung Journal of Medical Sciences*, *28*(8), 442–447.

Iqbal, M., Walpola, R., Harris-Roxas, B., Li, J., Mears, S., Hall, J., and Harrison, R. (2022). Improving primary health care quality for refugees and asylum seekers: A systematic review of interventional approaches. *Health Expectations*, *25*(5), 2065–2094.

Kardas, P., Lewek, P., and Matyjaszczyk, M. (2013). Determinants of patient adherence: A review of systematic reviews. *Frontiers in Pharmacology*, *4*, 91.

Kehlenbrink, S., Jobanputra, K., Reddy, A., Boulle, P., ... Ellman, T. (2023). Diabetes care in humanitarian settings. *Endocrinology and Metabolism Clinics*, *52*(4), 603–615.

Khdour, M.R., Awadallah, H.B., Alnadi, M.A., and Al-Hamed, D.H. (2020). Beliefs about medicine and glycemic control among type 2 diabetes patients: A cross-sectional study in West Bank, Palestine. *Journal of Primary Care & Community Health*, *11*. https://doi.org/10.1177/2150132720971919.

Krauskopf, K., Federman, A.D., Kale, M.S., Sigel, K.M., ... Wisnivesky, J.P. (2015). Chronic obstructive pulmonary disease illness and medication beliefs are associated with medication adherence. *COPD: Journal of Chronic Obstructive Pulmonary Disease*, *12*(2), 151–164.

Lyles, E., Burnham, G., Chlela, L., Spiegel, P., Morlock, L., LHAS Study Team, and Doocy, S. (2020). Health service utilization and adherence to medication for hypertension and diabetes among Syrian refugees and affected host communities in Lebanon. *Journal of Diabetes & Metabolic Disorders*, *19*, 1245–1259.

Mann, D.M., Ponieman, D., Leventhal, H., and Halm, E.A. (2009). Predictors of adherence to diabetes medications: The role of disease and medication beliefs. *Journal of Behavioral Medicine*, *32*, 278–284.

WHO (2024). Diabetes [Press release]. 14 November 2024. Available at: https://www.who.int/news-room/fact-sheets/detail/diabetes (Accessed 6 October 2025).

THREE

Working with agency: agency as a driver of continuity of HIV care among Ukrainian refugees fleeing to Denmark

Emilie Mai Anderberg, Marie Nørredam, and Morten Skovdal

When the war in Ukraine escalated in February 2022, millions of people were forced to flee their homes and cross borders, fearing for their lives and the continuity of their chronic disease care. Among them are Maria, Roman, Andrii, and Dmytro, four Ukrainian refugees living with human immunodeficiency virus (HIV), whose stories and quest for health have inspired this chapter. Their quest for HIV care represents an active and continuous pursuit to access and maintain healthcare services despite the uncertainties of forced displacement, HIV-related stigma, language barriers, and encountering unfamiliar healthcare systems. This quest goes beyond the mere act of seeking medical treatment; it involves a series of strategic, pensive, and sometimes desperate actions to ensure continuity of HIV care. Their stories reveal that accessing healthcare along migratory routes depends heavily on refugees' agentic capabilities and motivation to navigate and advocate for their health needs. Drawing on qualitative research methodologies, this chapter argues that agency is crucial in maintaining continuity of chronic disease care in displacement, especially when encountering new and different health systems. While this may work for some, it poses challenges for many others. Although it is essential to recognise the agentic capabilities of some refugees to self-care, agency to the extent we have observed must not be a prerequisite to access HIV care. Health and HIV services along migratory routes must be made more accessible for refugees.

Introduction

Globally, there are more than 115 million forcibly displaced persons (UNHCR, 2024). The war in Ukraine has displaced over 14 million people, seeking refuge both within Ukraine and beyond (IOM, 2024). Many have crossed borders to reach neighbouring countries, and others have continued their journey further into Europe. This situation has led to the separation of families, abandonment of homes, and restricted access to healthcare services, exacerbating numerous protection risks for the displaced people. The crisis in Ukraine has placed significant demands on health systems to address a multitude of health issues among the displaced, necessitating continuity of care and sustained access to medicines in Ukraine, in transit, and in destination countries (Health Policy Watch, 2022). Among these health challenges is the need for regular HIV treatment and services. This is underscored by reports, which estimate that up to 30,000 Ukrainians living with HIV, most of whom were receiving treatment, have been forcibly displaced across Europe since the onset of the war in February 2022 (ECDC, 2022).

The widespread need for HIV care among Ukrainian refugees underscores the fact that HIV continues to be a major global public health issue. Fortunately, with the broad availability of antiretroviral therapy (ART), it is now commonly managed as a chronic health condition (WHO, 2024). The ART regimen involves taking a daily combination of medications that suppress HIV and maintain immune function. When individuals consistently engage in care, adhere to their daily ART regimen, and maintain regular contact with healthcare services, they can achieve and sustain an undetectable viral load. This not only allows them to live long and healthy lives but also prevents the onward transmission of the HIV virus. However, inconsistent adherence can lead to drug resistance, reduced treatment effectiveness, and increased risk of progression to acquired immunodeficiency syndrome (AIDS).

Reflecting the urgency of these needs, global health actors have set ambitious targets to end AIDS as a public health threat by 2030 (UNAIDS, 2021; United Nations, 2024). Achieving this goal requires continuous and uninterrupted access to treatment for tens of millions of people in need of long-term care. Within this global framework, Ukraine plays a critical role. It is home to the second-largest HIV epidemic in Europe and Central Asia, with an estimated 1 per cent of the population living with HIV (UNAIDS, 2019). Prior to the war, the country was making significant progress in its national AIDS response, with an increasing number of people living with HIV receiving ART and successfully managing their health and well-being (UNDP, 2022). However, the realities of war and displacement complicate these efforts, posing unique challenges for displaced persons living with HIV. The potential disruptions they face, such as discontinuation or interruption of treatment, or late diagnosis, could have significant public health impacts.

War and armed conflicts have devastating effects on the health and well-being of all people involved, as well as on the social life within and surrounding the war-affected regions. Russia's aggression in Ukraine, including attacks on healthcare facilities, ambulances, and critical infrastructure, has severely compromised the availability of essential services and medications and created new crises within the health and social system (Khanyk et al, 2022; eyeWitness et al, 2023). Additionally, forced displacement or migration can act as a determinant of health, putting the physical, mental, and social well-being of refugees at risk (Abubakar et al, 2018; WHO, 2022). As individuals are displaced, cross international borders, and move from their countries of origin through transit to host countries, their health is shaped by the distinct conditions of each stage of their migratory journey (WHO, 2022). Factors like traumatic experiences, access to healthcare and social services, availability of shelter and food, social networks, logistical challenges, security conditions, stigma and discrimination, language barriers, cultural values, and social and migration policies can significantly impact their health and well-being (WHO, 2022; IOM, 2023). For those living with chronic diseases such as HIV, the breakdown of healthcare systems and the shortage of medication, coupled with forced displacement, can have a profound impact on their short- and long-term health.

This chapter explores qualitatively how a group of Ukrainian refugees navigated and managed their chronic disease care while living with HIV amid the challenges posed by forced displacement. It delves into how their agentic capabilities, with motivation acting as a foundational force, enabled them to overcome structural barriers and maintain continuity of care. Here, agency is understood as the capacity of individuals to actively manage their health by pensively making informed decisions, seeking out alternative resources, advocating for their specific health needs, and participating proactively in healthcare processes (Bandura, 1997, 2006; Renkens et al, 2022). In the face of war and forced displacement, the exercise of such agency may not only enable individuals to influence their health outcomes amid surrounding instability but also showcase their resilience and adaptability, empowering them to reshape their interactions with and expectations of healthcare systems globally.

Insights from Ukrainian refugees

This chapter draws upon a qualitative study that explored how refugees fleeing from Ukraine to Denmark maintained continuity of HIV care. The individuals involved, Maria, Roman, Andrii, and Dmytro, are Ukrainian refugees linked to HIV care in Denmark. They were aged between 25 and 50 years and had been living with HIV for durations ranging from three months to 21 years at the time of the interviews. They were selected using purposive sampling from four Departments of Infectious Diseases in Denmark to ensure a diverse representation of experiences related to their continuity of care. All four individuals have been given pseudonyms to protect their identities.

Semi-structured interviews were conducted between March and May 2023 to capture their lived experiences of navigating HIV care in Ukraine, through transit countries, and finally in Denmark, their country of destination. All interviews were conducted in either Russian or Ukrainian. With the aid of interpreters skilled in cultural sensitivity, language and cultural aspects were bridged, ensuring that the nuances of their experiences were thoroughly understood and respected. Data were analysed using NVivo 1.7.1 and thematic network analysis (Attride-Stirling, 2001). This approach allowed us to delve deeply into their personal stories. The findings uncover how Maria, Roman, Andrii, and Dmytro exercise agency, fuelled by motivation, in their quest for HIV care throughout their migratory journey. Their stories demonstrate how they navigate, adapt, and persist in securing their health needs despite various challenges, illustrating how individuals manage their chronic disease care amid displacement. The study was approved for ethical clearance by the Research Ethics Committee for the Faculty of Science and the Faculty of Health and Medical Sciences, University of Copenhagen.

Working with agency

This section examines how the agencies of Maria, Roman, Andrii, and Dmytro facilitate the effective management of their health needs during the distinct phases of pre-migration, transit, arrival, and integration in Denmark. Their stories reveal that exercising agency involves more than mere action; it encompasses motivation, derived from intentional, forward-thinking, self-regulatory, and reflective abilities that empower and encourage them to navigate complex healthcare systems and maintain continuity of HIV care. A key observation is that those who had been diagnosed most recently generally experienced greater challenges in navigating their new situation and maintaining motivation, especially due to fear of stigma and lack of social support. Those who had been living with HIV for a longer period had more experience with the illness, including previous periods without treatment, which gave them a more long-term perspective on the pros and cons of taking their medication and maintaining a stable condition.

Pre-migration phase: planning and preparedness in securing HIV treatment

In the pre-migration phase, Maria, Roman, Andrii, and Dmytro exemplified remarkable, forward-thinking, and proactive actions in securing their HIV treatment, even as the sudden experience of war threatened their stability. Their actions underscore their determination to maintain continuity of care amid the escalating crises. Yet, their resolve was immediately tested as they began their migratory journey.

Planning during times of conflict

On the evening before her evacuation, Maria was making an intentional effort to secure additional ART, fully aware that the journey ahead could severely disrupt her access to medication. Her anticipation of the unpredictability of fleeing a war zone motivated her to act. Maria recounted:

> I went to see my doctor and asked if it was possible to get any extra ART meds because we were about to

be evacuated the next day. The doctor said that at that point, they didn't have any stocks of meds [ART], and they didn't know when the meds would be delivered. So, I only had two months of therapy left, and that was it. I was happy to still have some ART while the area was being bombed. (Maria, 48)

Despite facing evacuation, Maria's motivation to maintain her health drove her to secure her medication. Similarly, Roman made a strategic decision to secure his ART supply before crossing borders, yet fleeing the conflict zone. His ability to think ahead and act deliberately led him to register at an HIV clinic in Kyiv to ensure he had enough medication to last throughout the uncertain period of his displacement: 'When I was leaving the occupied area, I was running out of medications [ART]. In Kyiv, I registered at an HIV clinic and got enough medication for six months more before leaving Ukraine' (Roman, 50).

By carefully planning their medical needs ahead of anticipated treatment disruptions, Maria and Roman made efforts to maintain their continuity of HIV treatment. As both faced medication shortages and restricted access to HIV clinics later in their migratory journey, their strategic planning proved essential in managing their treatment regimen.

Transit phase: choosing appropriate courses of action in seeking HIV care when crossing borders

During the transit phase, Maria, Roman, Andrii, and Dmytro navigated the complexities of crossing borders and seeking HIV care in unfamiliar environments, coping with the fear of HIV-related stigma, securing safe shelter, and handling constant uncertainty. Their stories underscore the power of personal drive and advocacy in maintaining care continuity while crossing borders.

CONTINUITY OF CARE

Advocating against HIV-related stigma

An essential component of their agency was demonstrated through their difficult decisions to disclose their HIV status to humanitarian workers. The profound psychosocial impact of stigma, stemming from the public's beliefs and negative attitudes as well as experiences of discrimination from healthcare workers in Ukraine, often leads to fear, shame, and isolation among all individuals, as Dmytro recalled: 'Imagine this scenario: When you come home to visit your family, they have set aside a separate bowl, a separate spoon, a separate dish for you, and they ONLY give it to you when you come to visit' (Dmytro, 48).

Such experiences, manifesting throughout their life course, highlight the burden of stigma that individuals living with HIV must continually navigate. Motivated by the need to maintain their health, they adapted their behaviour to access essential care, advocating fearlessly for their right to life-saving treatment, prioritising their health needs over the potential of facing stigma. This is exemplified by Maria:

> If it hadn't been for my 'fearlessness', I would not have access to ART today. I went into every office at the Red Cross and was not afraid to tell them that I have such and such a diagnosis [HIV], and need therapy [ART], or to be registered somewhere, or to be examined by a doctor. I asked, I stood, and I told them to their face. I was not afraid. (Maria, 48)

By strategically choosing when and with whom to share her HIV status, Maria demonstrated how she clearly understood her care needs, monitored her situation, balanced her options, and adapted her strategies to advocate for her health rights. Similarly, Dmytro exhibited willpower as he, to maintain continuity of HIV treatment, immediately communicated his medical needs upon reaching refugee camps: 'I had 3 months' worth of ART medication from Ukraine ... From the very first day I said that

I would need ART, and they promised they would give it to me at the camps. They never gave me anything' (Dmytro, 48).

His advocacy, fuelled by his battles with AIDS symptoms and the stigma he faced, drove a deep-seated awareness of the devastating impacts of treatment interruption. This personal context empowered him to confront and overcome the frequent delays and unmet promises that he encountered while navigating healthcare in unfamiliar territory.

Maria and Dmytro demonstrated self-directed actions by effectively managing their personal information about their HIV status while persistently seeking access to necessary care, though their efforts were ultimately unsuccessful. Driven by a strong motivation to maintain their health, they tackled the stigma and systemic obstacles from humanitarian organisations, including delays, unfulfilled commitments, and a lack of recognition for their proactive health management. Their ability to navigate the complexities of securing care in unfamiliar and precarious environments, without passively waiting for assistance, exemplifies their commitment to adapt and overcome challenges. Furthermore, their actions underscore the critical need for health systems to be flexible and responsive, recognise and support the agency of those they serve, and ensure continuous care amid the challenges posed by cross-border movements.

Arrival and integration phase: finding the motivation and energy to navigate a new healthcare system and reconnect with HIV services

Upon arrival in Denmark, Maria, Roman, Andrii, and Dmytro found themselves on a continuous quest to reconnect with HIV treatment by accessing HIV services in Denmark. Despite the Danish healthcare system offering free and high-quality treatment, they encountered various obstacles, including a lack of information about HIV services, complex pathways to care, and language barriers. Nonetheless, their reflective actions during this phase illustrate their relentless pursuit of the motivation and energy required to adeptly navigate a new healthcare system and successfully reconnect with HIV services.

Navigating care needs with motivation

Maria's repeated efforts to reconnect with HIV services exemplify the arduous tasks in navigating a new healthcare system. Despite facing setbacks, her unwavering determination drove her to advocate for her care needs. Maria describes her experience:

> In Denmark, I went through all the camps and Red Cross centres, one by one, asking for a doctor to take tests and decide on therapy [ART]. No one could help; they kept saying, 'We don't know, you don't have a yellow card yet [health insurance card].' I said to them: 'You must understand, ART is not just a headache pill; it's essential for my survival, and I have a child with me.' But no one cared, and I could sit and wait for a CPR number. Fortunately, I still had some of my medication. (Maria, 48)

She strategically challenged the system, keenly aware of the consequences of missing her ART. Faced with the critical situation of running out of medication, she considered taking extreme measures to draw attention to her urgent need for care: 'I thought that if I were too exhausted, if I became sick or something else happened, maybe then the medical and social workers would finally pay attention to me. I would finish what I had left of my ART, and then let things take their course' (Maria, 48).

Maria's persistence in seeking care underscores her deep commitment to her health goals, whatever it takes. She was forced to shift her strategy and sought personal contacts through online HIV groups across Europe, eventually connecting with a hospital worker in Denmark. This hospital worker played a pivotal role in fulfilling Maria's quest to reconnect with HIV services. Dmytro, facing the urgency of coming to the end of his ART supply, took decisive action to address his situation with the help of a Russian-speaking social worker:

> It came to the point that when I received a yellow card, I had only one pill left, and nothing had progressed. I called my social worker and informed him about my HIV status, and he finally contacted the family doctor. The next day, the doctor saw that I had only one pill left, he called a hospital in Copenhagen directly, and I went to get the medicine the next day. (Dmytro, 48)

Ultimately, his ability to leverage community resources played a significant role in facilitating access to HIV care and overcoming bureaucratic hurdles. Andrii, diagnosed with HIV three months after arrival, sought informal alternatives to formal HIV clinics while waiting for his health insurance card. He accessed care through Checkpoint, a free community-based clinic that provides anonymous and direct referrals, ensuring a smoother transition to necessary services. This was crucial in securing HIV care that met his needs for sensitivity and stigma-free entry into the healthcare system. Andrii reflected on the process: 'I came across Checkpoint one day, went in, and was directly referred to the hospital. When I was diagnosed with HIV it was overall okay, compared to if I had found out at home [in Ukraine], it would have been more difficult' (Andrii, 25).

After successfully reconnecting with HIV services, all individuals were satisfied with the treatment they received. However, they encountered significant communication challenges such as language barriers, a shortage of interpreters, and difficulties in addressing specific care needs, ultimately leading to delayed access to broader services. Additionally, their reluctance to disclose their HIV status widely made them hesitant to discuss their condition openly with many health professionals. Notably, the need for multiple disclosures in the Danish referral system proved to be a struggle. Roman illustrated this point:

> I feel comfortable with the Danish doctors, but the system here differs. In Denmark, the infectious disease doctor only handles infectious diseases and refers other issues to the general practitioner, who then refers to specialists. It would be easier to return to Ukraine for a health issue and come back to Denmark afterwards. (Roman, 50)

Despite these issues, Maria, Roman, Andrii, and Dmytro leveraged their health literacy to enhance communication with healthcare professionals. They maintained effective communication by focusing on a shared 'treatment language' centred around CD4 counts, symptoms, and ART regimens. This strategic use of medical terminology and knowledge not only facilitated their treatment continuity but also empowered them to be active participants in their care management.

Armed with a deep understanding of their HIV disease and the critical importance of maintaining continuous care, Maria, Roman, Andrii, and Dmytro navigated arduous pathways to care and communication challenges to reconnect with HIV care in Denmark successfully. Their quest is a testament to their ability to carefully evaluate each situation, adapt, seek out, utilise available networks, and take deliberate actions to advocate for their health needs in an unfamiliar environment. Additionally, their persistent energy and motivation, derived from personal contexts and health goals, proved to be a critical element fuelling their agency and bridging gaps created by structural barriers. Moreover, their narratives highlight the crucial need for healthcare systems to adopt person-centred care tailored to the needs and expectations of displaced populations.

A cross-border quest for health

For individuals managing chronic conditions like HIV, the journey through forced displacement is not just a physical relocation; it's an ongoing, multifaceted quest for health. This quest unfolds across the phases of pre-migration, navigating transit, integrating into new healthcare systems, and sometimes returning. However, literature concerning healthcare needs and chronic disease management of displaced populations during all phases of the migratory journey is underrepresented (WHO, 2022). This chapter contributes to the limited evidence and demonstrates that each phase requires not only available health services but also the capacity of some individuals to access, seek, engage with, and benefit from these services to maintain chronic disease care and contribute to healthy communities. The experiences of Maria, Roman, Dmytro, and Andrii illustrate the crucial role of agentic capabilities and motivation in maintaining the continuity of HIV care amidst the challenges of displacement.

Being forcibly displaced from their homes due to conflict or violence, individuals living with chronic conditions must anticipate their short- and long-term healthcare needs, often with great unpredictability. Securing ART before crossing borders was a crucial first step for Maria and Roman in managing their disease needs and avoiding interruption in treatment. Planning, however, is not a simple task. A review found that both disruption of medication supplies and limited access to providers in conflict zones were associated with perceived worsening of disease and critically impacted the continuity of treatment among internally displaced persons (Cantor et al, 2021). Strengthening national health systems' preparedness and response to ensure that essential medications and services reach internally displaced populations promptly can mitigate some of these burdens and improve health outcomes for those most at risk.

During the transit phase, displaced individuals must contend with the uncertainty of crossing borders and seeking chronic disease care in unfamiliar environments. For Maria and Dmytro, their personal drive and proactive engagement with humanitarian workers became a lifeline in their self-care management when humanitarian responses did not meet their care needs. While the individuals in this chapter took agency for their care management, humanitarian responses must recognise the displaced persons with limited ability, energy, or motivation to take on an active or co-creating role to ensure continuity of chronic care. Furthermore, humanitarian response during transit should prioritise access to chronic disease care that meets the diverse needs of displaced populations (WHO, 2023; Aljadeeah et al, 2025).

Upon arrival in their host country, refugees must navigate a new healthcare system and adjust their strategies to meet their chronic care needs. Despite the Danish healthcare system offering free services to Ukrainian refugees, barriers such as limited information, language differences, and fear of HIV-related stigma remain challenges. Arora et al identified similar barriers to HIV care linkage and long-term treatment engagement (Arora et al, 2021). Nonetheless, with motivation and by leveraging informal community networks and their HIV literacy, Maria, Roman, Andrii, and Dmytro enhanced communication and trust with healthcare professionals, ensuring successful reconnection with HIV services. Building on this agency, a Danish study found that when healthcare systems create safe and encouraging environments, it motivates refugees to open up and take an active role in coproducing their health (Radl-Karimi et al, 2022). National health systems must ensure that services are accessible, responsive, and tailored to the diverse needs of refugee populations. Moreover, their pursuit of health across borders highlights a critical deficiency in global healthcare systems: the lack of comprehensive, accessible services throughout all stages of migration that ensure continuity of chronic disease management and address the diverse needs of displaced populations..

Conclusion

This chapter has illustrated the critical role of agency in maintaining the continuity of HIV care for Ukrainian refugees like Maria, Roman, Andrii, and Dmytro. Their narratives demonstrate how agency, fuelled by motivation, acts as a driver enabling individuals to navigate and overcome substantial barriers when formal health systems do not meet their needs. Due to their active role in their own care management, they successfully reconnected with HIV care in Denmark, ensuring both short-term and long-term health and well-being.

While acknowledging the agentic capabilities of some refugees is essential, we must ensure that such agency is not a prerequisite for accessing HIV care. Ensuring that chronic health and HIV services along migratory paths are available and made more accessible to all refugees is vital to ensure continuity of care. Health professionals and humanitarian workers should actively engage with and respond to the unique needs of displaced persons in the design and implementation of health services. Moreover, by strengthening health systems to be more adaptive and responsive to the needs of displaced populations, we can create more inclusive and equitable health services that cater to the unique challenges faced by displaced individuals. This alignment with differentiated service delivery and people-centred principles is key to achieving global health targets and ensuring no one is left behind.

References

Abubakar, I., Aldridge, R.W., Devakumar, D., … Zimmerman, C. (2018). The UCL–Lancet Commission on Migration and Health: The health of a world on the move. *The Lancet (British edition)*, *392*(10164), 2606–2654. doi:10.1016/S0140-6736(18)32114-7

Aljadeeah, S., Hosseinalipour, S.-M., Khanyk, N., Szocs, E., … Veizis, A. (2025). Healthcare provision for displaced people in transit: Analyses of routinely collected data from INTERSOS clinics at the Ukrainian border with Moldova and Poland. *Journal of Migration and Health*, *11*, 100287. doi:https://doi.org/10.1016/j.jmh.2024.100287

Arora, A.K., Ortiz-Paredes, D., Engler, K., Lessard, D., … Lebouché, B. (2021). Barriers and facilitators affecting the HIV care cascade for migrant people living with HIV in Organisation for Economic Co-operation and Development countries: A systematic mixed studies review. *AIDS Patient Care STDS*, *35*(8), 288–307. doi:10.1089/apc.2021.0079

Attride-Stirling, J. (2001). Thematic networks: An analytic tool for qualitative research. *Qualitative Research: QR*, *1*(3), 385–405. doi:10.1177/146879410100100307

Bandura, A. (1997). *Self-efficacy: The exercise of control.* W H Freeman/Times Books/Henry Holt & Co.

Bandura, A. (2006). Toward a psychology of human agency. *Perspectives on Psychological Science*, *1*(2), 164–180. doi:10.1111/j.1745-6916.2006.00011.x

Cantor, D., Swartz, J., Roberts, B., Abbara, A., ... Smith, J. (2021). Understanding the health needs of internally displaced persons: A scoping review. *Journal of Migration and Health*, *4*, 100071. doi:10.1016/j.jmh.2021.100071

ECDC (2022). Operational considerations for the provision of the HIV continuum of care for refugees from Ukraine in the EU/EEA.

PHR (2023). *Destruction and Devastation. One Year of Russia's Assault on Ukraine's Health Care System.* Physicians for Human Rights. https://phr.org/our-work/resources/russias-assault-on-ukraines-health-care-system/ (Accessed 6 October 2025)

Health Policy Watch (2022). As Ukrainians flee, WHO stresses importance of lifesaving NCD care for refugees and migrants. Available at: https://healthpolicy-watch.news/ncd-care-for-refugees/ (Accessed 6 October 2025).

IOM (2023). EMM2.0 Handbook: Health and migration. Available at: https://emm.iom.int/handbooks/health-and-migration (Accessed 6 October 2025).

IOM (2024). Ukraine & Neighbouring countries: Two years of response. UN Migration. Available at: https://www.iom.int/sites/g/files/tmzbdl486/files/documents/2024-02/iom_ukraine_neighbouring_countries_2022-2024_2_years_of_response.pdf (Accessed 6 October 2025).

Khanyk, N., Hromovyk, B., Levytska, O., Agh, T., Wettermark, B., and Kardas, P. (2022). The impact of the war on maintenance of long-term therapies in Ukraine. *Front Pharmacol*, *13*. doi:10.3389/fphar.2022.1024046

Radl-Karimi, C., Nielsen, D.S., Sodemann, M., Batalden, P., and von Plessen, C. (2022). 'When I feel safe, I dare to open up': Immigrant and refugee patients' experiences with coproducing healthcare. *Patient Education and Counseling, 105*(7), 2338–2345. doi:https://doi.org/10.1016/j.pec.2021.11.009

Renkens, J., Rommes, E., and van den Muijsenbergh, M. (2022). Refugees' agency: On resistance, resilience, and resources. *International Journal of Environmental Research and Public Health, 19*(2). doi:10.3390/ijerph19020806

UNAIDS (2019). Global AIDS Monitoring 2019: Ukraine summary. Available at: https://www.ecoi.net/en/file/local/2038369/UKR_2020_countryreport.pdf (Accessed 6 October 2025).

UNAIDS (2021). Global AIDS Strategy 2021–2026: End nequalities. *End AIDS*. Available at: https://www.unaids.org/en/resources/documents/2021/2021-2026-global-AIDS-strategy (Accessed 6 October 2025).

UNDP (2022). AIDS and war: How Ukraine is combatting HIV/AIDS in 2022. Available at: https://www.undp.org/ukraine/news/aids-and-war-how-ukraine-combatting-hiv/aids-2022 (Accessed 6 October 2025).

UNHCR (2024). Refugee data finder. Available at: https://www.unhcr.org/refugee-statistics/insights/explainers/forcibly-displaced-pocs.html (Accessed 6 October 2025).

United Nations (2024). The 17 Goals | Sustainable Development. Available at: https://sdgs.un.org/goals (Accessed 6 October 2025).

WHO (2022). World report on the health of refugees and migrants. Available at: https://www.who.int/publications/i/item/9789240054462

WHO (2023). Promoting the health of refugees and migrants: Experiences from around the world. Available at: https://iris.who.int/server/api/core/bitstreams/2b4e46e8-5358-4c65-b0ba-5ecf10d7c141/content (Accessed 6 October 2025).

WHO (2024). HIV and AIDS. Available at: https://www.who.int/news-room/fact-sheets/detail/hiv-aids (Accessed 6 October 2025).

PART II

Social relations

FOUR

Working through community structures: the role of community health workers in cardio-metabolic disease care in Bidibidi, Uganda

Tania Aase Dræbel, Bishal Gyawali, Dricile Ratib, Rita Nakanjako, Esther Kalule Nanfuka, Emmanuel Raju, David Kyanddodo, and Morten Skovdal

This chapter examines how community health workers (CHWs) support refugees with diabetes and hypertension in accessing health services and engaging in self- and social care. Despite limited resources, CHWs perform three critical roles: 1. Relational Work: CHWs connect with the community, facilitate communication with healthcare staff, help patients re-engage with services, advocate for patients, and act as intermediaries. 2. Healthcare Work: CHWs monitor and screen for illnesses, refer complex cases, promote health, deliver medication, monitor adherence, and follow up with patients. 3. Community Engagement Work: CHWs assess community conditions, engage in sensitisation, and mobilise efforts. These three types of work are crucial to maintaining the continuity of care for refugees with chronic conditions. Our findings underscore the importance of CHWs and the need to integrate them into the formal healthcare system.

Introduction

The global burden of non-communicable diseases is growing. This is also the case in Uganda, home to more than 1.6 million refugees (WHO, 2024), many of whom struggle to access diagnosis, treatment and care for non-communicable diseases, including diabetes and hypertension. Mobility and migratory movements can exacerbate poor health, delay diagnoses, and contribute to the discontinuation of treatment and care. Refugees also face challenges when it comes to accessing treatment services and informal care for non-communicable diseases in their resettlement communities. While much work has gone into unpacking barriers to non-communicable disease treatment, such as stigma and discrimination (Dong et al, 2021), language barriers (Mashaba et al, 2024) and difficulties accessing medication (Tusubira et al, 2020), comparatively little has been done to explore pathways to treatment and care for non-communicable diseases more broadly. Against this background, we explore the mediating and facilitating role of CHWs in supporting refugees' continuity of care for diabetes and hypertension in Bidibidi, the largest refugee settlement in sub-Saharan Africa. We approach care continuity as the continued engagement with formal treatment and care services and the ability to sustain health through self-care and social support.

To improve access to healthcare, particularly in rural areas, the Ministry of Health in Uganda introduced the Village Health Team programme in 2001 as part of the National Minimum Health Care Package (MoH, 2015). A village health team member is a volunteer community health worker. Integrated into the healthcare system at the entry level (Health Centre I), they have become the first point of contact for healthcare delivery in community-based primary healthcare programmes nationwide (MoH, 2010). The CHWs that form part of a village health team receive monetary and non-monetary incentives. They typically lack formal training but receive localised instruction specific to the communities they serve, and topics often depend on the source of funding (Agarwal et al, 2021). CHWs in Uganda have significantly improved access to different health services, resulting in reductions in child mortality (Brenner et al, 2011) and the control of infectious diseases (Lewin et al, 2010).

CHWs' involvement in managing diabetes and HTN is relatively new and remains understudied (Chang et al, 2019). Research conducted in humanitarian settings (Slama et al, 2017) or in South Asia (Jafar et al, 2020; Gyawali et al, 2021) suggests that CHWs can raise awareness, counsel and monitor health status, as well as enhance communication between healthcare providers and patients. CHWs have also been assigned roles in implementing e-health interventions for individuals living with diabetes or hypertension, for instance, in Argentina (He et al, 2017) and Iran (Bozorgi et al, 2021). A study in Uganda found that non-communicable diseases (NCD) prevention and control can benefit from incorporating CHWs in health education, community mobilisation, screening, and referral of patients to health facilities (Musoke et al, 2021). The authors also stress the importance of strengthening CHWs' knowledge about NCDs. In a study among American patients with diabetes, Collinsworth et al (2013) found that CHWs play essential roles in helping patients understand their conditions better, which, according to the authors, enhances their adherence to treatment plans. The authors also note that CHWs help patients navigate the complexities of diabetes care by offering medication assistance and access to community resources. The authors call for further research to understand the roles and challenges of CHWs in caring for people living with chronic conditions across various health system contexts. We take heed of this call and explore the work done by CHWs in the Bidibidi refugee settlement to support the continuity of care for refugees living with diabetes and hypertension.

About the study

Design and location

This exploratory, qualitative study was conducted in 2023 in the Bidibidi refugee settlement, located in the Yumbe district of the West Nile region in Uganda. Bidibidi hosts approximately 198,184 forcibly displaced persons, mainly from South Sudan (UNHCR, 2024). It is the largest refugee settlement camp in Uganda and the second largest in the world. Villages in the Bidibidi settlement have CHWs, mirroring the Ugandan health structure.

Participants for the study were selected among the CHWs in Bidibidi. A purposive sampling method was employed to select participants based on the following criteria: 1. South Sudanese refugees residing in Bidibidi for at least six months; 2. actively involved as CHWs; 3. able to read, write, and speak English; and 4. willing to provide verbal informed consent.

The study included ten CHWs, each working in Bidibidi's five zones. All CHWs were South Sudanese men aged between 22 and 39 from the Greater Equatorial region. They fled to Uganda in 2016. All of them had completed the equivalent of O-levels, with four completing A-levels. One CHW had received training as a teacher, while another had experience in animal husbandry. Six CHWs were married with children, while four were single without children.

Data collection and analysis

The first author interviewed all the participating CHWs, guided by a structured topic guide drafted in English focusing on CHWs' potential for ensuring care continuity for diabetes and hypertension. Interviews were conducted via online platforms (Zoom and Skype) and lasted 50 to 100 minutes.

The interviews were recorded and transcribed verbatim by the first author. The data were analysed using inductive thematic analysis to identify common themes and discrepancies within the data. Following the approach outlined by Braun and Clarke (2006), we conducted a thematic analysis as an iterative process in six steps. As an initial step, the first author familiarised themselves with the data by listening to the interviews and reading the transcripts. In the second step, codes were generated from the interviewees' statements. The coding of statements led to the third step, which involved generating themes from the codes. In the fourth and fifth steps, themes were reviewed, defined, and named. In the sixth step, examples supporting each theme were selected from the interview material. Through this process, we arrived at three main themes: 1. CHWs' relational work, 2. Healthcare work, and 3. Community work. Participation was voluntary, and participants could withdraw from the study at any time.

Findings

Relational work
Bridging relations between the community and healthcare workers

Contact between the community and the health facility requires literal and figurative translation. Few in the community can communicate in English, and few of the healthcare workers are familiar with the languages the refugees speak. Some healthcare workers have limited knowledge of languages such as Kawka, Lugbara, or Luo, but not enough to communicate effectively with patients. When patients visit a health facility, healthcare workers expect them to bring someone who can translate on their behalf, ideally a family member. CHWs may also be solicited because they know the services and the system and can speak the same language as the healthcare workers. CHWs can, therefore, play a crucial role in facilitating communication between patients and healthcare workers.

CHWs can act as 'go-betweens' when issues occur between patients and healthcare workers. For instance, when a patient refuses to go to the health facility to get her drugs because she has repeatedly experienced that the clinic staff told her to go and buy her treatment at the private clinic. As exemplified by William, a CHW, it is common for CHWs to encourage patients to continue seeking care at the health centre:

> They [clients] say: 'You go there, and you come back, minus the drug.' They are told that if they have the money, they had better go to buy the drugs at the clinic; even if they don't have the money, they are being told they should go and buy. This is not all right! However, as CHWs, we must advise clients to visit the health clinic'. (William, 39, CHW)

CHWs explain that they can help patients re-engage with the health clinic when patients have had a 'fall-out' with a healthcare worker. For instance, if a patient arrives late for an appointment for follow-up or for getting medication or seeks health services outside the days scheduled for follow-up and treatment of diabetes and hypertension, healthcare workers may rebuke patients:

> One client went to the health clinic to get her drugs. However, she was late. She tried to approach the doctor, but the doctor was harsh and asked her, 'Why are you late? I have my own things [to look after], so I will not see you today. You come back another day!' So the client went home without her medicines. (John, 22, CHW)

CHWs can act as the *advocate* of persons living with diabetes and/or hypertension who depend on receiving food adapted to their dietary needs. During a meeting with district representatives and the Office of the Prime Minister, Phillip, a CHW, voiced his concern: 'I want to know, is there going to be any [food] support for these clients? [with diabetes or hypertension]' (Phillip, 38, CHW).

A few CHWs experienced healthcare workers' attitudes as an obstacle to patients going to the health centre for treatment.

CHWs can act as intermediaries to bridge the understanding between patients and healthcare workers. Some patients and their families believe in traditional healers and herbalists for diabetes treatment, leading them to seek care outside health facilities. CHWs can act as negotiators between patients or their families and health facilities to prevent patients from suffering from complications of uncontrolled diabetes and/or hypertension.

Some CHWs successfully guide patients towards prescribed treatment, but some patients or their family prefer alternative options to the prescribed treatment:

> Sometimes we get negative feedback from the clients about the health clinic. They [clients] have their activity and are busy, so if you refer them, they don't want to go to the health clinic. If I write a referral to the health clinic, some people can say 'no,' they refuse going there. The first thing they will tell me is: 'you go there and then you come back, minus the drug, even when you have the money, there is no drug. So, you better go to the [private] clinic that is better'. Even when they don't have the money, you can get the treatment from the [private] clinic. They [clients] feel bad about going to the health clinic; they believe that they will not get the drugs. (William, 39, CHW)

Healthcare work
Screening and monitoring, incl. for diabetes and hypertension

Screening and monitoring for diabetes and hypertension are not a part of CHWs' formal responsibilities. Some CHWs follow patients diagnosed with multiple conditions, including hypertension. Few CHWs have access to machines to measure blood pressure. At patients' request, CHWs can measure blood pressure:

So sometimes, we borrow the blood pressure machine at the health clinic and go to the client. We are not trained in this. I am doing this because in South Sudan, I did health work, and when I came here, I became close with my health assistant, and he told me about this [prevalence of high blood pressure], so I felt that I should do something about this in my community. (Simon, 28, CHW)

CHWs use machines for measuring blood pressure provided by an organisation, which in 2020 initiated a project aimed at monitoring the health of pregnant women in the community. As part of the project, CHWs in two out of five zones were enrolled, trained and equipped with BP machines. When the project was discontinued in 2021, five blood pressure machines were left with CHWs.

Referral to the health centre, including for diabetes and hypertension

CHWs identify and manage common illnesses in the community. Cases that cannot be managed in the community are referred to relevant health facilities. CHWs' work also involves following up on and monitoring cases of common illnesses. CHWs need to know when and whom to refer and follow up on the referral to ensure the patient is taken to the nearest health facility.

If they [community] have a health problem, they come to me. I have been doing integrated health management for under 5 years. I treat children below 4 years and 11 months; cases like cough, diarrhoea and malaria are managed in the community. If it [health problem] is within my capacity. If it is not within my capacity, I refer to the health facility.

CHWs also refer patients with diabetes and hypertension to the health clinic, even though they have not been trained to do so. Sometimes, patients are unable to go themselves or find a family member to take them to the health clinic. In such situations, health clinics have an ambulance that can transport the patient free of charge to either the clinic or the referral hospital in Yumbe. A CHW can contact the health clinic and request that the facility send an ambulance. However, CHWs may also accompany patients to the health centre and, for instance, arrange transportation to and from the facility.

Health promotion and education, including for diabetes and hypertension

CHWs reported promoting health and offering health education to patients. CHWs explained that they routinely provide education and counselling on infant and childhood illnesses, pregnancy-related conditions, and ante- and post-natal care. During household visits, interviewees are to observe and offer advice on health behaviours, health practices, hygiene, health conditions, and nutrition.

CHWs also mentioned that they may be approached by community members who have signs and symptoms of diabetes and/or hypertension. For instance, one CHW recounted a situation where he helped clarify and provide counsel to the community member: 'Now I have experience. If people share their symptoms like dizziness, thirst with me, I can tell them to do this and that, or that may be due to sugar or pressure' (John, 22, CHW).

A few CHWs describe that they promote and educate about diabetes and hypertension:

> People ask me, 'What are the symptoms of sugar and pressure? How does a person feel if s/he has sugar?' I tell them, 'You have a greater urge to urinate, you get hungrier.' Then I ask them if they have such symptoms. If they say yes, I refer them to the health centre, explaining that I don't have any extra kits. They get confused about

where to go, and what can I say instead of telling them to go to the medical or hospital? If there are leftover kits, I will give them to some people. But I wish I could tell all of them, 'let's check your sugar then'. (John, 22, CHW)

CHWs may also be approached to provide advice on prescribed medicines with undesirable side effects:

I follow a man, he is 58 years old, he has diabetes and high BP at the same time. So when I do follow up, I always go to check on him, whether he has his drugs and whether he is improving. At times, he may have pain, and he may have signs and symptoms that make him feel uncomfortable. He told me about his problems, like frequently having to urinate during the night, and food, the food he is not supposed to eat, and he was also telling me that some drugs were given to him that make him feel a headache. So, I advised him to return to the health clinic, and then the doctor or clinical officer could change the medicine. When he feels unwell, he calls me, and I can advise him on what is necessary. (Jonas, 26, CHW)

Other CHWs may be asked for advice on how to take the prescribed medication:

Sometimes, clients are given the drugs without counselling on how to take the drugs or the side effects. They ask me about the drugs. I can also teach about the side effects and benefits of taking the drugs. And I know that if the condition worsens, I will have to refer them to the health centre. (John, 22, CHW)

John also considers that offering 'psycho-social and moral support' constitutes an important part of his responsibilities to persons living with chronic conditions, such as diabetes and/or hypertension.

Delivering prescribed medication to patients with chronic conditions

CHWs can ensure continuity of care by delivering medication to patients who cannot transport themselves to the health facility. This includes patients who are blind, paralysed, in a wheelchair, or too weak to walk the distance to the health clinic. Roads may also be flooded during the rainy season. Interviewees described fetching medicines for patients, either on an ad-hoc basis or as part of their routine: 'My neighbour, she cannot move because of her legs; she has wounds, so I bring her the medicine' (Jonas, 26, CHW).

Monitoring adherence

CHWs routinely monitor adherence to treatment for tuberculosis and HIV. Frequently, patients will discontinue their prescribed treatment. CHWs know that stress related to forced displacement may explain why persons on directly observed therapy (for tuberculosis) and/or antiretroviral therapy (for HIV) disengage with treatment and care-seeking. CHWs also know about the importance of following up on patients who are on treatment for chronic conditions: 'The most important thing is the follow-up' (Phillip, 38, CHW) CHWs are also aware of the limits of their work in case patients are too stressed to adhere to treatment:

> As a CHW, the only thing you can do is to counsel them on the importance of staying on their medicine. Talk to them and advise and counsel them to take their medication. When someone is stressed and at the same time is not eating, some tend to stop taking their medication. So, when we give them the drugs, they keep the medication inside, but they are not swallowing it. So, we can talk and say: This drug will keep you alive; if you don't take this, the disease will kill you. (Simon, 28, CHW)

CHWs follow-up on patients who discontinue their treatment, as explained by Jonas, a CHW:

> We also follow up on clients with chronic illnesses like cases of high blood pressure and diabetes. We remind the patient of the date she is supposed to go and get her refill [of medicine at the health clinic] or to check on the person on how she is doing. (Jonas, 26, CHW)

Community engagement work
Recording and examining conditions in the community

CHWs participate in the surveillance and identification of community health and social issues, such as malnutrition or violence against women and children.

CHWs are also tasked with activities contributing to information management and planning community health interventions. They map the community, maintain the community registrar, and submit summary reports, analysing the information recorded in the register. CHWs are responsible for keeping village health records up to date, promoting health (often focused on malaria, tuberculosis and HIV), checking for signs of malnutrition, following the health and progress of pregnant and newborn mothers, as well as reporting and referring community members to health facilities.

Some CHWs, trained on blood pressure and blood sugar measurement, reported recording and examining pregnant women for high blood pressure or community members with signs or diagnoses of diabetes or hypertension.

Community sensitisation and mobilisation

'We do all this work in the community with the community' (John, 22, CHW).

When community leaders, partner organisations, or health clinics need to communicate with the community, they enlist the help of CHWs to convey the message. Health workers also ask CHWs to mobilise the community when they have an announcement about health services available at the nearest health centre, such as 'health talks' on diabetes, hypertension, HIV counselling, testing, surveys, and childhood immunisation.

CHWs also organise village-wide health activities that benefit the entire community, such as cleaning areas near the communal water supply, repairing and constructing latrines, or removing trash. CHWs use mobilisation to engage the community in decisions about health and social issues. The assumption is that when people are involved, they are also in a better position to make informed decisions about matters affecting their lives and their community.

Discussion

This study has explored the work done by CHWs to ensure continuity of care for refugees affected by diabetes or hypertension in the Bidibidi refugee settlement. In summary, CHWs play a critical role in ensuring access to health for children under five and pregnant mothers. CHWs do regular home visits, including identification and management of common illnesses. CHWs also follow up on patients treated with directly observed therapy and antiretroviral therapy, and support patients in maintaining care continuity for diabetes and hypertension. Altogether, CHWs ensure the community's access to health services. In this study, we identify three dimensions of CHWs' work that are essential to care continuity. CHWs' relational work, healthcare work, and community work ensure continuity of care for diabetes and hypertension. CHWs are eager to learn and are highly motivated to expand the range of their services to include raising awareness about diabetes and hypertension, screening, monitoring, and managing patients with diabetes and/or hypertension. However, CHWs are challenged by a lack of training on prevention and management of diabetes and hypertension, knowledge gaps among patients about diabetes and hypertension prevention and treatment, a lack of medicines in the health clinics due to stock-outs, overcrowded and understaffed health clinics, and no screening and monitoring for diabetes and hypertension in the community. This finding is supported by a qualitative study among CHWs in Uganda (Chang et al, 2019) and a study about managing hypertension in rural Uganda (Stephens et al, 2020).

We find that CHWs ensure care continuity by establishing and maintaining relationships with patients and their families. Other research among Ugandan CHWs exemplifies that CHWs provided with training can link the community to healthcare for diabetes and hypertension (Mugisha and Seeley, 2021). CHWs' relational work reduces the social distance between the community and Bidibidi's healthcare workers. CHWs' shared life experiences with the refugee community they serve are reinforced by their social proximity in Bidibidi, and these two factors combined may lead CHWs to be better attuned to their community's needs for self-care, social care, and healthcare. This finding resonates with research on how CHWs may have an advantage in establishing relations of trust, which in turn is a condition for health communication and support (Knowles et al, 2023) and the community's access to health services (Ndambo et al, 2022).

A key finding of this study is that the healthcare work of CHWs is essential for maintaining care continuity in patients with diabetes and/or hypertension. CHWs bridge the community to the healthcare system, facilitating access to health services. Research from other contexts has shown that CHWs reduce barriers to accessing health services by inviting communities to health-promoting activities, health education, and support to navigate the health system (Ngcobo et al, 2022). In a study conducted among people living with diabetes in Venezuela, Babagoli et al (2021) examined the informal role of CHWs in an environment with a pluralistic health system. They conclude that CHWs can 'leverage their intimate knowledge of local practices to provide decision-making support to patients'.

Studies from both high-income and low- and middle-income countries have shown the role of community health workers in increasing awareness and access to health services in rural areas (Javanparast et al, 2018). CHWs provide services at the household level, enabling them to reach the most vulnerable and underserved individuals in a community who may otherwise struggle to access care (McCollum et al, 2016).

CHWs play a key role in engaging the community in health-related activities. Other studies have shown how community involvement in health promotion can ensure the relevance and effectiveness of health programmes. Health-enabling community engagement promotes collaboration between healthcare providers and service users, enhancing the understanding of health needs and access barriers to healthcare services (LeBan, Kok, and Perry, 2021). Our findings show that CHWs engage the community in various health-related activities. As deomnstrated by Ngcobo et al (2022) and Murphy et al (2021), CHWs ability to engage with the community and build trust is key to health promotion and improving access to care. A study by Khatri et al (2023) shows that community engagement may improve decision-making processes and health by factoring in social determinants of health. Yet, Khatri et al underline that there are political, cultural, and organisational factors which may influence community engagement. Hence, the need to carefully consider both the barriers to and the potential for this engagement, which may lead to more efficient and sustainable health programmes. CHWs can be central to health-enabling community engagement, but as some studies have shown, different contexts require different approaches to this form of community engagement. Therefore, there is a need to continue exploring and adapting approaches to this type of community engagement that are relevant and efficient for the community.

The voluntary work of CHWs, including visiting households, facilitating transportation, delivering medications, and assisting non-English speakers during consultations, appear essential to care continuity. CHWs act as a 'go-between' between the community and healthcare workers. Health services and the community rely on CHWs to bridge this gap. This finding is supported by Perry et al (2019), who have shown that the CHWs' shift between roles of 'insider', 'outsider', and 'intermediaries' allows the CHWs to link the community to health clinics. CHWs being 'insider' in the community is a challenge as the CHWs feel compelled to share their meagre resources. Perry et al argue that ongoing supervision, additional training and teamwork with other CHWs are key to balancing their diverse roles. Being both insiders and outsiders, CHWs are required to set clear boundaries for their work. The community or health workers do not always understand or respect such boundaries. Becoming a CHW involves navigating expectations and power dynamics, which can lead to disappointment and entanglement in complex power relations. CHW efforts to overcome healthcare barriers in Bidibidi can inadvertently lead to tensions, potentially eroding their social credibility and legitimacy if not managed effectively.

According to our research, many CHWs 'go the extra mile' to address obstacles to care continuity for diabetes and hypertension, including stock-outs of government medicines, patients' irregular attendance at health facilities, and irregular treatment among patients (Stephens et al, 2020). CHWs utilise their resources, including time, phone credit, and money, to assist patients in attending consultations at health facilities, obtaining medications, and reaching patients and their relatives through social media or other platforms.

While it is well established that CHWs play an essential role in linking patients to health facilities, this study has demonstrated how this is achieved through largely hidden relational work. This work comprises three key activities: facilitating communication between the community and health facility staff; monitoring and screening for common illnesses, including diabetes and hypertension; and recording and assessing conditions within the community while engaging the community in sensitisation and mobilisation efforts.

Research on CHWs highlights the crucial role of CHWs in bridging the community to health services. This work may be largely invisible, yet it is crucial for the continuity of care.

Conclusion and recommendations

CHWs are essential to the upkeep of healthcare in Bidibidi. Their integration into the formal health system is crucial for the prevention and management of common illnesses, as well as the continuity of care for hypertension and diabetes. Our study contributes to existing knowledge by demonstrating how the CHWs' largely invisible work within their community helps reduce the gaps between self-care, social care, and formal healthcare.

The CHWs manage despite many obstacles, such as scarcities in both personnel and other supplies, including access issues for monitoring and early diagnosis, but this is unsustainable. For CHWs to realise their potential in diabetes and hypertension care continuity, they require training, equipment, transportation means, and compensation for their time. The minimum equipment for CHWs should include electronic BP machines for screening and monitoring, bicycles for mobility, and phone credit to facilitate communication between patients, the community, and health workers.

To address community needs, one CHW per village could be selected for health education and promotion, focusing on diabetes and hypertension. Community engagement should include dialogues, radio talk shows, outreaches, and integrated programmes.

If CHWs are to create awareness, screen, monitor, and manage diabetes and hypertension, care and follow-up need to be strengthened at other levels of the health system. This requires added financing for diabetes and hypertension programmes, health workforce training, continuous monitoring, and evaluation and improved diagnostic equipment at referral levels.

Acknowledgements

We want to thank the participants who generously shared their time, experiences, and insights as part of this study. This work was funded by the Novo Nordisk Foundation (ref. NNF21OC0062473).

References

Agarwal, S., Abuya, T., Kintu, R., Mwanga, D., Obadha, M., Pandya, S., and Warren, C.E. (2021). Understanding community health worker incentive preferences in Uganda using a discrete choice experiment. *Journal of Global Health*, *11*, 07005.

Babagoli, M.A., Nieto-Martínez, R., González-Rivas, J.P., Sivaramakrishnan, K., and Mechanick, J.I. (2021). Roles for community health workers in diabetes prevention and management in low-and middle-income countries. *Cadernos de saude publica*, *37*(10), e00287120.

Bozorgi, A., Hosseini, H., Eftekhar, H., Majdzadeh, R., … Ashoorkhani, M. (2021). The effect of the mobile 'blood pressure management application' on hypertension self-management enhancement: A randomized controlled trial. *Trials*, *22*(1), 413.

Braun, V. and Clarke, V. (2006). Using thematic analysis in psychology. *Qualitative Research in Psychology*, *3*, 77–101.

Brenner, J.L., Kabakyenga, J., Kyomuhangi, T., Wotton, K.A., … Kayizzi, J. (2011). Can volunteer community health workers decrease child morbidity and mortality in southwestern Uganda? An impact evaluation. *PloS One*, *6*(12), e27997.

Chang, H., Hawley, N.L., Kalyesubula, R., Siddharthan, T., Checkley, W., Knauf, F., and Rabin, T.L. (2019). Challenges to hypertension and diabetes management in rural Uganda: a qualitative study with patients, village health team members, and health care professionals. *International Journal for Equity in Health*, *18*(1), 38. doi:10.1186/s12939-019-0934-1

Collinsworth, A.W., Vulimiri, M., Schmidt, K.L., and Snead, C.A. (2013). Effectiveness of a community health worker-led diabetes self-management education program and implications for CHW involvement in care coordination strategies. *The Diabetes Educator*, *39*(6), 792–799.

Dong, R., Leung, C., Naert, M.N., Naanyu, V., … Edelman, D. (2021). Chronic disease stigma, skepticism of the health system, and socio-economic fragility: Qualitative assessment of factors impacting receptiveness to group medical visits and microfinance for non-communicable disease care in rural Kenya. *PloS One*, *16*(6), e0248496.

Gyawali, B., Sharma, R., Mishra, S.R., Neupane, D., Vaidya, A., Sandbæk, A., and Kallestrup, P. (2021). Effectiveness of a female community health volunteer–delivered intervention in reducing blood glucose among adults with type 2 diabetes: An open-label, cluster randomized clinical trial. *JAMA Network Open*, *4*(2). doi:10.1001/jamanetworkopen.2020.30921.

He, J., Irazola, V., Mills, K.T., Poggio, R., … Bazzano, L.A. (2017). Effect of a community health worker-led multicomponent intervention on blood pressure control in low-income patients in Argentina: A randomized clinical trial. *JAMA*, *318*(11), 1016–1025.

Jafar, T.H., Gandhi, M., De Silva, H.A., Jehan, I., … Khan, A.H. (2020). A community-based intervention for managing hypertension in rural South Asia. *New England Journal of Medicine*, *382*(8), 717–726.

Javanparast, S., Windle, A., Freeman, T., and Baum, F. (2018). Community health worker programs to improve healthcare access and equity: Are they only relevant to low-and middle-income countries? *International Journal of Health Policy and Management*, *7*(10), 943.

Khatri, R., Endalamaw, A., Erku, D., Wolka, E., Nigatu, F., Zewdie, A., and Assefa, Y. (2023). Continuity and care coordination of primary health care: A scoping review. *BMC Health Services Research*, *23*(1), 750.

Knowles, M., Crowley, A.P., Vasan, A., and Kangovi, S. (2023). Community health worker integration with and effectiveness in health care and public health in the United States. *Annual Review of Public Health*, *44*(1), 363–381.

LeBan, K., Kok, M., and Perry, H.B. (2021). Community health workers at the dawn of a new era: 9. CHWs' relationships with the health system and communities. *Health Research Policy and Systems*, *19*, 1–19.

Lewin, S., Munabi-Babigumira, S., Glenton, C., Daniels, K., … Scheel, I.B. (2010). Lay health workers in primary and community health care for maternal and child health and the management of infectious diseases. *Cochrane Database Syst Rev*, *2010*(3), Cd004015. doi:10.1002/14651858.CD004015.pub3

Mashaba, R.G., Seakamela, K.P., Mbombi, M.O., Muthelo, L., … Ntimana, C.B. (2024). Recognition of language barriers in comprehending non-communicable disease management among rural elderly people in the DIMAMO surveillance area: a case of AWI-Gen participants. *BMC Public Health*, *24*(1), 2782.

McCollum, R., Gomez, W., Theobald, S., and Taegtmeyer, M. (2016). How equitable are community health worker programmes and which programme features influence equity of community health worker services? A systematic review. *BMC Public Health*, *16*, 1–16.

MoH (2010). *Village Health Team: Strategy and Operational Guidelines*. Ministry of Health, Uganda.

MoH (2015). *Village Health Team Strategy and Operational Guidelines*. Ministry of Health, Uganda.

Mugisha, J.O. and Seeley, J. (2021). 'We shall have gone to a higher standard': Training village health teams (VHTs) to use a smartphone-guided intervention to link older Ugandans with hypertension and diabetes to care. *AAS open Research*, *3*, 25.

Murphy, J.P., Moolla, A., Kgowedi, S., Mongwenyana, C., … Pascoe, S. (2021). Community health worker models in South Africa: A qualitative study on policy implementation of the 2018/19 revised framework. *Health Policy and Planning*, *36*(4), 384–396.

Musoke, D., Atusingwize, E., Ikhile, D., Nalinya, S., ... Gibson, L. (2021). Community health workers' involvement in the prevention and control of non-communicable diseases in Wakiso District, Uganda. *Globalization and Health*, *17*, 1–11.

Ndambo, M.K., Munyaneza, F., Aron, M., Makungwa, H., Nhlema, B., and Connolly, E. (2022). The role of community health workers in influencing social connectedness using the household model: A qualitative case study from Malawi. *Global Health Action*, *15*(1), 2090123.

Ngcobo, S., Scheepers, S., Mbatha, N., Grobler, E., and Rossouw, T. (2022). Roles, barriers, and recommendations for community health workers providing community-based HIV Care in Sub-Saharan Africa: A review. *AIDS Patient Care and STDs*, *36*(4), 130–144.

Perry, S., Fair, C.D., Burrowes, S., Holcombe, S.J., and Kalyesubula, R. (2019). Outsiders, insiders, and intermediaries: Village health teams' negotiation of roles to provide high quality sexual, reproductive and HIV care in Nakaseke, Uganda. *BMC Health Services Research*, *19*, 1–12.

Slama, S., Kim, H.-J., Roglic, G., Boulle, P., ... Tonelli, M. (2017). Care of non-communicable diseases in emergencies. *The Lancet*, *389*(10066), 326–330.

Stephens, J.H., Alizadeh, F., Bamwine, J.B., Baganizi, M., ... Mukiza, J. (2020). Managing hypertension in rural Uganda: Realities and strategies 10 years of experience at a district hospital chronic disease clinic. *PloS One*, *15*(6), e0234049.

Tusubira, A.K., Akiteng, A.R., Nakirya, B.D., Nalwoga, R., Ssinabulya, I., Nalwadda, C.K., and Schwartz, J.I. (2020). Accessing medicines for non-communicable diseases: Patients and health care workers' experiences at public and private health facilities in Uganda. *PloS One*, *15*(7), e0235696.

UNHCR (2024). Uganda: Refugees and nationals by district. Available at: https://data.unhcr.org/en/country/uga (Accessed 23 May 2024): UNHCR.

WHO (2024). Refugee and migrant health system review: Challenges and opportunities for long-term health system strengthening in Uganda. World Health Organization.

FIVE

Working alongside interpreters: optimising communication for continuity of care for refugees in Uganda

Rita Nakanjako, Esther Kalule Nanfuka, Morten Skovdal,
Susan Reynolds Whyte, and David Kyaddondo

Effective patient-provider communication is crucial for continuity of care; however, language barriers often impede effective communication in refugee settings. While using interpreters is a common strategy to address this, little research has explored the dynamics of interpreter-mediated communication in low-resource refugee contexts. This chapter examines the limitations and strategies for optimising interpreter-mediated patient-provider communication in a rural Ugandan refugee settlement. Drawing on in-depth interviews with refugees, interpreters, and healthcare providers at Nyumanzi Health Centre III, the chapter highlights how interaction, relational, contextual, and interpreter competence issues constrain effective communication. Optimising interpreter-mediated communication for continuity of care requires multipronged approaches to build capacities, manage expectations, improve working conditions, and foster trust among patients, providers, and interpreters in resource-limited humanitarian settings.

Introduction

Continuity of care depends heavily on good patient-provider communication. In refugee settings, good patient-provider communication is often impossible due to language barriers (Kavukcu and Altıntaş, 2019). Language barriers have been reported to adversely affect the continuity of care for refugees and immigrants with chronic conditions, as they have special long-term healthcare needs (Kotovicz et al, 2018). They are associated with interruptions in treatment adherence and poor chronic disease management (Pandey et al, 2021), loss to follow-up, and poorer health outcomes (Rasi, 2020). Therefore, addressing language barriers is critical in the provision of healthcare for refugees who usually have no realistic opportunity to acquire the language of the host country before their flight (Kletečka-Pulker et al, 2018).

Using interpreters is one of the most prominent strategies for addressing language barriers in providing healthcare to refugees. Healthcare systems in refugee destination countries typically have formal mechanisms in place to promote the routine use of trained interpreters. In Uganda, interpreters are recruited as part of the essential healthcare workforce in health facilities in refugee settlements and reception centres (WHO, 2024). Interpreters serve as a conduit, transmitting information between the healthcare provider and their refugee patients (Dysart-Gale, 2005). Their role involves rendering in one language literally what has been said in the other without any additions, omissions, editing, or polishing (Roat et al, 1997). As such, interpreters are trained to use the first-person singular, creating the impression of dyadic physician–patient communication and minimising their presence (Hsieh, 2006). However, in practice, interpreters play a more active role.

In refugee healthcare, interpreters assume multifaceted roles that enhance the quality of provider-patient interactions and communication. Besides their primary role of translation, interpreters have been found to provide emotional support to refugee patients (Hsieh, 2008). In addition, interpreters play a cultural consultancy role (Gartley and Due, 2017), providing not only language translation, but also the mediation of cultural or ethnic norms and understandings (Miller et al, 2005). In this way, interpreters play a critical role in assisting refugee patients and healthcare providers in developing culturally feasible treatment plans (Hsieh and Hong, 2010).

While interpreters are critical in the provision of healthcare to refugees and other non-native speakers (Heath et al, 2023), they are not a panacea for language barriers between patients and providers. Their use in the provision of healthcare to refugees and immigrants is associated with several limitations, which encompass: not always being available (MacFarlane et al, 2020); loss of context and emotional meanings of information (Raval, 2003); anonymity, bias, confidentiality and misinterpretation challenges (MacFarlane et al, 2020); mistrust, which constrains the self-disclosure and openness of refugee patients (Jiménez-Ivars and León-Pinilla, 2018); as well as incidents where interpreters overstep their expertise and role boundaries (Hsieh and Hong, 2010). These limitations can undermine trust in interpreter-mediated patient-provider communication.

Despite the undeniable challenges inherent in working alongside interpreters to provide healthcare to refugees, their role remains critical. Evidence suggests that when healthcare providers and refugee patients lack proficiency in a common language, the use of interpreters has a positive impact on the quality of care and clinical outcomes for refugee patients (Boylen et al, 2020). This underlines the need to optimise interpreter-mediated patient-provider communication to augment the quality of care provided to refugees. Despite this, little research addresses the question of how to optimise the use of interpreters in refugee patient healthcare, particularly in the global south and humanitarian contexts. This chapter explores the limitations of, and strategies for optimising, interpreter-mediated patient-provider communication in a rural refugee settlement in Uganda from the perspectives of patients, providers and interpreters.

About the study

Study design

An exploratory design was employed to gain new insights into the limitations of interpreter-mediated patient-provider communication in humanitarian settings and the measures that can be taken to optimise it. A qualitative approach was employed to obtain in-depth accounts of participants' personal experiences with interpreter-mediated patient-provider communication. This provided insights into their perceptions regarding the limitations of interpreter-mediated patient-provider communication in the context of refugee healthcare and how it can be optimised.

Study location and participants

The study participants included six adult (18 years and above) male and female refugee patients with hypertension and diabetes seeking care from Nyumanzi Health Centre III (HCIII). Other participants included interpreters (n=6) and healthcare providers (three clinical officers, and five nurses) working with refugee patients at the health facility. All were sampled purposively based on their experience and engagement with interpreter-mediated patient-provider communication in refugee healthcare settings.

Nyumanzi HCIII is a public facility serving refugees based in the nearby Nyumanzi Settlement and Reception Centre and the surrounding host population. While the facility is officially a Health Centre II, its capacity has been scaled up to that of a Health Centre III by the United Nations High Commissioner for Refugees (UNHCR) partner for health, Medical Teams International (MTI), to accommodate the large refugee population. Nyumanzi HCIII employs seven interpreters, who are contractual staff of MTI and receive a monthly salary of UGX305,000 (USD83). These interpreters serve an average population of 150 outpatients and 17 inpatients daily. The interpreters are recruited through a formal process that begins with the placement of an advertisement calling for refugees with the requisite qualifications, such as a minimum education level of primary seven, proficiency in English, and the dominant languages used by refugees in the targeted settlement, and proceeds through shortlisting, interviews, and the selection of successful candidates. The selected candidates are oriented about their role before being assigned health facility duties. The orientation typically takes five days and focuses not only on the principles of interpretation but also on counselling, communication, and mediation of patient-provider interactions. The orientation is conducted by the in-charge (a clinical officer) and selected staff of the health facility. The interpreters support various departments at the facility, including outpatient, maternity, laboratory, consultation rooms with clinical officers, and pharmacy on a rotational basis.

The settlement and the health facility are in the Northwestern District of Adjumani in Uganda. Adjumani is the second-largest refugee-hosting district in the country. As of August 2024, Adjumani had 225,096 refugees, which was 12.9 per cent of the total refugee population in Uganda (UNHCR, 2024). Nyumanzi is the largest settlement in Adjumani district, hosting an estimated 50,000 refugees. Most (90 per cent) of the refugees in Nyumanzi Settlement are South Sudanese of the Dinka ethnic group, although not all refugees in Nyumanzi speak Dinka. When we conducted the study, the ethnic diversity of the patient population of Nyumanzi HCIII had been compounded by the influx of refugees from Sudan and some ethnic Nuer South Sudanese, hosted in the nearby Nyumanzi

Reception Centre. The literacy levels of refugees in Uganda are generally low, with an estimated 75 per cent considered illiterate (UNHCR, 2023).

Data production and analysis

We held four group interviews (GIs), one with each category of participants. The group interviews enabled each participant to share their personal experiences while reflecting on one another's ideas (Bell, 2012). This provided rich insights into the participants' views about the limitations of interpreter-mediated patient-provider communication and how it can be optimised in refugee healthcare services. Data were collected between August 2023 and July 2024. Interviews were conducted at Nyumanzi HCIII and moderated by two of the authors. The interviews were conducted using a topic guide, which allowed participants to express their views and narrate their experiences in their own words. The interpreters and healthcare providers were interviewed in English, while the patients were interviewed in a mix of English and Dinka. Two peer researchers attached to the CONTINUITY research project served as interpreters during patient interviews. The group interviews lasted an average of 90 minutes.

Data management and analysis

All the interviews were audio recorded, translated into English where necessary, and transcribed verbatim. They were then word-processed and imported into NVivo12, a qualitative data analysis software package, for coding and management. Data analysis was conducted thematically. The process involved reading transcripts of data on each participant several times while coding the relevant sections, paragraphs, and words according to categories and themes that emerged from the data or were identified from the literature.

Ethical considerations

Ethical approval was obtained from the Makerere University School of Social Sciences Research and Ethics Committee (MAKSSREC03.23652) and the Uganda National Council for Science and Technology (SS1843ES). All participants gave written informed consent, were informed about the study, and were assured of confidentiality.

Characteristics of study participants

The patients constituted equal numbers of males and females. All of them were living with hypertension and/or diabetes. Their ages ranged from 37 to 64 years. Only one had attained some formal education. All were South Sudanese refugees of the Dinka ethnic group and had lived in Uganda for ten or more years. Only one spoke English, with the rest only proficient in Dinka and/or Arabic and Nuer.

All the providers (nurses and clinical officers) were Ugandans from the northern part of the country. Most (four) were from the Acholi ethnic group, followed by Madi (three) and one Alur. Their ages ranged from 28 to 44 years. While all the clinical officers were male, the nurses constituted three females and two males. They had served at Nyumanzi HCIII for an average of four years. None of the providers spoke Dinka or any other native language of the refugee community.

All the interpreters were South Sudanese refugees of the Dinka ethnic group. Like the patients, all the interpreters were residents of Nyumanzi Settlement. Most (four) were female. Their age ranged from 26 to 35 years. All had attained some level of formal education. One had completed Senior 4, two stopped in Senior 2, one stopped in Senior 3, one stopped in Primary 7, while one had obtained a certificate in sociology. They all spoke Dinka and English, with some also speaking Arabic and Kiswahili. All had considerable experience interpreting patient-provider communication in refugee healthcare, having served for an average of eight years.

Perceived limitations of interpreter-mediated patient-provider communication

Doubt among providers and patients

Both patients and providers reported that they often questioned the accuracy of interpretation. While interpreters are expected to communicate exactly what the patient or provider says without changing the meaning, health workers reported incidents where interpreters expressed the patients' words in technical terms, raising doubts about the accuracy of interpretation and ultimately the reported concern of the patient.

> the interpreter may not use the exact words of the patient and may make some adjustments. For example, a patient may say I have chest pain then the interpreter tells you the patient says he has epigastric pain. Sometimes, you may find that we ask patients to touch the area where they feel the pain. (GI with Clinical Officers)

In addition, doubt was evoked when the duration of the interpretation was significantly shorter than the time the patient used to explain their problem. Providers generally expected the interpretation to take a similar amount of time. However, sometimes, the interpretations were relatively brief, making providers believe that something was lost in translation.

> I always have doubts ... because sometimes a patient speaks for a long time, and the interpreter only makes a very brief statement. As a provider, I doubt whether he interprets the patient's words 100%. I expect that when the patient speaks for a long time, the interpreter

must also talk for a long time. He is supposed to take at least 75% of the time the patient has taken, but sometimes, halfway through, the interpreter is done. (GI with Nurses)

Interpreters attributed the reported inconsistencies in the duration of interpretation to incompatibilities between the native languages of refugees and English. For instance, it was indicated that lengthy statements in Dinka could be expressed in a few English words: 'in Dinka, you may find very many words, and when you express them in English, it is only one word. If a patient says a lot, then you mention 2 to 3 words, there will be doubt that you have not interpreted correctly' (GI with interpreters).

Doubt about the accuracy of interpretation was mainly triggered for the patients when the treatment plan did not meet their expectations. This often led to patients being dissatisfied with the quality of care they received.

We don't understand English... We have some doubts. When we talk to the doctor, then in the end, the medicine they give us is not what we expected. We think that maybe the interpreters did not interpret our words well. Also, if our blood tests are done and we get the right medicine, we trust that the interpreter did well. But we suppose the interpreters did not do well when they write out medicine without running tests. (GI with patients)

Confidentiality and trust concerns

Providers and interpreters reported confidentiality and trust issues arising from interpreters and patients being refugees who live in the same community. It was indicated that patients with sensitive and stigmatised conditions, such as reproductive health ailments, found it difficult to open up in the presence of interpreters, some of whom were close relatives, because they did not trust them to keep their issues confidential.

> Some of these interpreters are related to the patients; they may be in-laws, distant relatives, or neighbours. This may affect the way the patient opens up about their condition. Fortunately, NCDs are not stigmatised like HIV ... Sometimes we have sensitive issues that require privacy. ... the patient may not find it comfortable for the interpreter to be there. But because they have no choice, they go ahead and share, but occasionally you find some don't, especially the young people ... So, mostly confidentiality issues. (GI with Clinical Officers)

In some cases, the distrust and discomfort were associated with the gender of the interpreter. Patients were generally uncomfortable opening up about sensitive issues to interpreters of the opposite sex, with women and girls particularly affected. Women and girls in the Dinka community are socialised to fear men. Therefore, they are more likely to be uncomfortable sharing sensitive issues in the presence of male interpreters.

> The major concern is about confidentiality because interpreters stay together with the patients in the community. So, when patients have sensitive illnesses for example, a problem on the vulva or penis, they find difficulty disclosing when the interpreter is there. These interpreters are either females or males. Sometimes this person may be of the opposite sex to this interpreter, and this person may be coming from the same block, and the person may fear that this interpreter may reveal their issue to the community ... This is common among women because women fear men. (GI with Nurses)

In this regard, interpreters may be considered a barrier to effective patient-provider communication.

Concerns about bias

Interpreters reported that refugee patients commonly accused them of being biased and siding with Ugandan health workers when the treatment plans did not meet the patients' expectations or desires. The patients' accusations were rooted in the belief that interpreters, being 'one of them', should advocate for their interests rather than advance the agendas of health workers who were Ugandan and therefore 'outsiders'.

> These people [patients] accuse us of being biased. If we explain to them what the doctor said, they say we are siding with them. Arguments emerge, for example, when the doctor prescribes coartem [oral medicine] instead of an injection that the patient wants. They [patients] believe that the interpreters are siding with doctors who are Ugandans, yet, being South Sudanese like them, they should side with them. In other words, interpreters should support them [patients] to get that injection but now they are siding with the doctor to tell them to take tablets. (GI with interpreters)

Misrepresentation of information

Health workers reported that interpreters occasionally misrepresented providers' and patients' communication, leading to distorted responses. These incidents were attributed to interpreters limited medical knowledge, fear of consulting, and poor listening skills.

> you may ask a particular question, for example, 'Are you having a headache?' The response you will get from the interpreter is that the patient said he is vomiting, but that is not what you asked. This shows that sometimes they don't listen attentively. (GI with Clinical Officers)

> I had a scenario where the patient was prescribed amoxicillin, which is supposed to be taken 8-hourly, and it was written clearly on the dispensing envelope. It was indicated as tds [medical terminology for 3 times a day], not the usual 2 times 3. This interpreter did not understand the instructions and feared coming and inquiring. He just told the patient that you are going to take this medicine once a day. (GI with Nurses)

These incidents highlight the importance of interpreters possessing not only language proficiency but also strong interpersonal and other soft skills.

Increased consultation and patient waiting time

Interpretation was reported to increase individual patient consultation time, with effects on waiting time. Providers observed that interpretation often doubled or even tripled the time needed to review one patient. This not only increased their workload but also slowed down the rate at which patients were seen, necessitating that they wait longer.

> Because interpreting has to take place, you end up consuming a lot of time seeing your patients. ... the interpreter talks, then the patient talks and again through the interpreter, back to you. This increases the time spent on one patient. You may have like 20 hypertensive patients to review, assuming you planned to spend 5 minutes on each, you may end up spending 10 to 20 minutes or even 30 minutes ... This increases our workload; you have to put in more time, but it also means that the other patients wait longer. (GI with Clinical Officers)

Moreover, difficulties in finding enough interpreters for the ethnically diverse population of South Sudanese refugees from both the settlement and reception centre meant that, occasionally, two people were required to interpret from one local language to another, then English and vice versa. This further increased the time spent on one patient.

> you find scenarios where you need 2 interpreters. Like when we get patients who don't speak the dominant language, like Dinka. Here, most interpreters know Dinka, Arabic and English. But we sometimes get patients from the reception centre who speak Nuer, especially the new arrivals. In that case, we look for someone who knows Nuer and Dinka but may not speak English well. That person interprets the patient's communication to Dinka, then our interpreter interprets it into English for the doctor. They will then interpret the doctor's response from English to Dinka, then Dinka to Nuer back to the patient. (GI with Clinical Officers)

Too many patients, few interpreters

Interpreters complained about an excessive workload that compromised their effectiveness. It was indicated that each interpreter handled an average of 50 patients daily, some requiring more time to understand the provider's instructions. It was not uncommon for providers to request interpreters to engage patients further to help them understand their communication. Several of these encounters were emotionally draining for the interpreters, as the patients were often complex, argumentative, and sometimes abusive. The interpreters noted that the heavy workload wore them out and affected the accuracy of their work.

> We are few, and the patients are many. Each of us handles about 50 people a day. By the end of the day, we are tired. Sometimes it is hard to convince the patients of what the doctor has said. The doctor tells you to use your words

to make this patient understand. So, you talk and even take more time. They argue with you, don't listen to you, you explain to them their illnesses, and they don't accept what you are telling them. They can even abuse you. That process is draining; you get tired and annoyed because the person doesn't understand, even if you use your own language. This affects our accuracy. (GI with Interpreters)

Poor professional practice

Participants cited incidents of unprofessional conduct among interpreters. These included nepotistic tendencies, where interpreters flouted the health facility's first-come, first-served policy to get their close relatives treated first, and rudeness towards patients. Such unprofessional practices contributed to spoiling relationships among providers, patients, and interpreters and ultimately undermined the quality of care provided.

> A patient can come late to the clinic, but the interpreter wants you to see them first. This may be their relative or a neighbour. Yet the policy is first-come, first-served. This will affect the service provided. You will find people unhappy, bickering in the line. This affects the quality of services we provide to our clients. (GI with Clinical Officers)

Approaches for optimising interpreter-mediated communication for continuity of care

Study participants proposed several approaches to address the identified limitations as explained later.

Mentorship of interpreters

Mentorship of interpreters was underlined as a key strategy that can augment interpreter-mediated patient-provider communication in a refugee setting. The providers noted that mentorship is relevant in teaching interpreters how to build rapport with patients. One way is mentorship on how to handle patients, building rapport with them, and engaging in social interaction (GI with Clinical Officers).

Patients also raised the importance of training interpreters to build rapport with service users. They argued that this would create a positive health-seeking environment, encouraging them to visit the health facility and ultimately facilitating continuity of care. 'Interpreters should be trained on how to handle patients. When a patient arrives, they should be made to feel comfortable before they see the doctor. If they handle us well, it will encourage us to return to the health centre for treatment' (GI with Patients).

Additionally, providers argued that mentorship should include teaching them medical terminologies, as several interpreters have low formal education levels, while others have no prior knowledge of the medical field. This limited medical knowledge leads some interpreters to misinterpret prescriptions: 'Interpreters need to be given basic medical instructions and terminology. Yes, mainly the interpretation of the prescription, because sometimes they give incorrect instructions to patients regarding the prescribed medicine' (GI with the Nurse).

Interpreters' mentorship was also deemed imperative due to the dynamism of the medical field. Novel diseases emerge every day, making constant training and retraining of interpreters a necessity. Providers noted that interpreter training should include health information that spans all departments, as interpreters are rotated throughout the health facility. They emphasised that the training should also provide interpreters with information about the common ailments dealt with at the facility.

> The mentorship should cut across, for example, if it's about the laboratory, they need to know: ... What are the requirements? What do we need in the laboratory?

> What are the common tests done in the laboratory? It then moves to maternity and everywhere. Regular mentorship for them is very important. These interpreters are qualified in different things, and they are now in the health sector. Some are senior 4 leavers, others did some training in business, so they are not familiar with these medical terminologies. Additionally, the medical world is constantly evolving with new diseases emerging every day, which these interpreters need to be aware of in order to support us in doing a good job. (GI with Nurses)

Interpreters supported the need for mentorship as a means of overcoming their unfamiliarity with medical information.

Increasing the number of interpreters to serve in different departments

Providers and interpreters advocated for increasing the number of interpreters to cover each department of the health facility. They contended that having more interpreters would lower the patient-interpreter ratio, which is currently high because of the large number of refugees served by Nyumanzi HCIII.

> The interpreter-patient ratio is very high. We have 7 interpreters, but … 2 mainly support the nutrition department. Then, for the general patients, we have 5 remaining. It becomes difficult to cover all the departments because one person has to be off duty, and somebody might be on annual leave. We usually have only 3 on the ground, so it isn't easy. (GI with Clinical Officers)

Recruitment of multilingual interpreters and balancing of genders during selection

Providers advocated for recruiting multilingual interpreters and balancing gender during their selection. Having interpreters who speak multiple languages would ease communication and make health service provision more efficient. At the same time, gender balance would allow patients to access an interpreter of their choice, enabling them to freely discuss sensitive health conditions.

> There is a need to recruit interpreters who speak many languages. This would ease service provision, especially in cases where we get patients who speak languages other than English and Dinka. This can be supplemented by balancing the gender of the recruited interpreters. This would give all patients a chance to get an interpreter of their choice. If a patient is uncomfortable with a female interpreter and needs a male one, the centre should have enough male interpreters to choose from and vice versa. (GI with Clinicians)

Discussion

Our results show that limitations of interpreter-mediated patient-provider communication in refugee healthcare settings of Uganda encompass an interplay of interaction and relational problems, contextual issues, and constraints related to competencies and conduct of interpreters (MacFarlane et al, 2020). Most of the identified limitations centred on trust, undermining the confidence of both patients and providers in interpreter-mediated communication. Therefore, optimising interpreter-patient-provider communication in the context of refugee healthcare demands multiple strategies to address the various shortcomings to close the confidence gap emanating from distrust of interpreters.

Interpretation in medical settings requires broad knowledge and skills beyond speaking two or more languages fluently (Kletečka-Pulker et al, 2018). Language competence, basic medical knowledge, attitudes, communication skills, and professional ethics are critical for effective interpretation in medical settings (Tribe and Morrissey, 2014). In humanitarian settings where patient loads and levels of distress are high (Pandey et al, 2021), interpreters need stress management and counselling skills. This necessitates that training for interpreters incorporates both technical aspects (including their roles and functions, basic medical knowledge, and counselling and communication skills) and soft skills (including emotional intelligence, professional ethics, stress management, and self-care). While interpreters' understanding of medical terminology may increase the risk for distortion of patients' communication by replacing it with medical jargon, this can be minimised by reiterating their basic function as neutral conduits of patient–provider information.

In Uganda, the generally low levels of education among refugee interpreters necessitate a more practice-oriented training approach, utilising techniques such as role-playing, case studies, video recordings, discussions, and reflection sessions, to enhance understanding and skills acquisition. Effective training and mentorship can help minimise inefficiencies in interpretation that adversely affect the quality of care and working conditions, increasing consultation and waiting times for patients as well as working hours for both interpreters and providers (Heath et al, 2023). The training may further strengthen the confidence healthcare providers and patients have in the quality of interpretations.

Healthcare providers could also benefit from training on how to work alongside and relate to interpreters who are neither professional nor medical interpreters. For instance, providers need tips on how to rephrase terminologies and restate words (Rajiv et al, 2021), as well as to make a conscious effort to ask the interpreter about phases of the communication that may not be captured in the immediacy of the literal translation (Raval, 2003), to reduce the possibility of misunderstanding, misattribution, and miscommunication. In addition, language training on the basic vocabulary of the refugee community's languages can be beneficial, especially in the Ugandan context, where refugees tend to be settled according to their ethnic background. This can reduce miscommunications between providers and patients about symptoms that lead to misdiagnosis or miscommunications after a correct diagnosis (Espinoza and Derrington, 2021). Besides, learning the basic expressions of the patient's language will increase the level of trust and confidence between the patient and provider (Raval, 2003), as well as assist in bolstering a good operational relationship with the interpreters. Providers typically use body language and response length as indicators for identifying mismatches in interpretation (Gartley and Due, 2017). This study shows that such mismatches may stem from incompatibilities between the native languages of refugees and those of their host country. Therefore, knowledge of basic expressions in the dominant languages of refugees may help healthcare providers to recognise such mismatches and maintain their trust and confidence in the interpreters.

The provider-interpreter mutual expectations must be clarified before they start conducting a healthcare encounter, with some basic rules agreed upon (Sleptsova et al, 2014). Similarly, patients should always be informed and reminded about the roles assigned to interpreters to manage their expectations and prevent misunderstandings and conflicts. This could be done before every interpreter-mediated patient-provider encounter or during the education sessions provided to NCD patients on clinic days. It is not uncommon for interpreters to be blamed when patients receive unwelcome information through them, as they are assumed to have the power to affect the provider's decision (Jiménez-Ivars and León-Pinilla, 2018). Overall, refugees tend to regard interpreters as advocates because they share a culture and language (Tribe and Morrissey, 2014). From the patients' perspective, interpreters' roles transcend the neutral conduit, transmitting information between the provider and patient (Dysart-Gale, 2005), to more proactive ones of patient advocate and cultural broker (Hsieh, 2006). Since conceptions of interpreters' roles are generally fluid (Sleptsova et al, 2014), patients' role expectations of interpreters may not match the roles the host country health system assigns them. Clarifying the roles of interpreters to patients can help to harmonise their role expectations of interpreters and increase their trust and confidence in them.

Increasing the number of interpreters, while factoring in gender considerations, can enhance the interpreter-mediated patient-provider health-seeking experience by providing more choice for both patients and providers. It can also help to reduce the workload for interpreters to acceptable limits. Given the rising number of refugees and migrants in Africa and the inevitable need for communication and mediation across language barriers, interpreters are crucial for facilitating communication in these linguistically and culturally diverse contexts (Moser-Mercer et al, 2021). However, this will require additional resources, which necessitates the engagement of both the donor (UNHCR and its implementing partners for health) and the government of Uganda, which owns most of the health facilities providing care for refugees.

Conclusion

Optimising interpreter-mediated patient-provider communication for continuity of care in low-resource humanitarian settings requires collaborative efforts between healthcare providers and interpreters. Proactive steps are needed to address the critical limitations that impede the quality of this communication. A multipronged approach that builds capacities, manages expectations, and improves the working conditions of both providers and interpreters is ideal. Crucially, this approach must also build trust and confidence within the patient-provider-interpreter triad. With close collaboration between healthcare providers and interpreters, the continuity of care for refugee patients can be significantly improved, even in low-resource humanitarian settings.

Acknowledgement

We want to thank the participants who generously shared their time, experiences, and insights as part of this study. This work was funded by the Novo Nordisk Foundation (ref. NNF21OC0062473).

References

Bell, B. (2012). Interviewing: A technique for assessing science knowledge. In S.M. Glynn and R. Duit (Eds) *Learning Science in the Schools* (pp 347–364). Routledge.

Boylen, S., Cherian, S., Gill, F.J., Leslie, G.D., and Wilson, S. (2020). Impact of professional interpreters on outcomes for hospitalized children from migrant and refugee families with limited English proficiency: A systematic review. *JBI Evidence Synthesis*, *18*(7), 1360–1388.

Dysart-Gale, D. (2005). Communication models, professionalization, and the work of medical interpreters. *Health Communication*, *17*(1), 91–103.

Espinoza, J. and Derrington, S. (2021). How should clinicians respond to language barriers that exacerbate health inequity? *AMA Journal of Ethics*, *23*(2), 109–116. https://doi.org/10.1001/amajethics.2021.109

Gartley, T. and Due, C. (2017). The interpreter is not an invisible being: A thematic analysis of the impact of interpreters in mental health service provision with refugee clients. *Australian Psychologist*, *52*(1), 31–40.

Heath, M., Hvass, A.M.F., and Wejse, C.M. (2023). Interpreter services and effect on healthcare – a systematic review of the impact of different types of interpreters on patient outcome. *Journal of Migration and Health*, 7, 100162.

Hsieh, E. (2006). Conflicts in how interpreters manage their roles in provider-patient interactions. *Social Science & Medicine*, *62*(3), 721–730.

Hsieh, E. (2008). 'I am not a robot!' Interpreters' views of their roles in health care settings. *Qualitative Health Research*, *18*(10), 1367–1383.

Hsieh, E. and Hong, S.J. (2010). Not all are desired: Providers' views on interpreters' emotional support for patients. *Patient Education and Counseling, 81*(2), 192–197.

Jiménez-Ivars, A. and León-Pinilla, R. (2018). Interpreting in refugee contexts. A descriptive and qualitative study. *Language & Communication, 60*, 28–43.

Kavukcu, N. and Altıntaş, K.H. (2019). The challenges of the health care providers in refugee settings: A systematic review. *Prehospital and Disaster Medicine, 34*(2), 188–196.

Kletečka-Pulker, M., Parrag, S., Drožđek, B., and Wenzel, T. (2018). Language barriers and the role of interpreters: A challenge in the work with migrants and refugees. In T. Wenzel and B. Drožđek (Eds), *An uncertain safety: Integrative health care for the 21st century refugees* (pp 345–361). Springer.

Kotovicz, F., Getzin, A., and Vo, T. (2018). Challenges of refugee health care: Perspectives of medical interpreters, case managers, and pharmacists. *Journal of Patient-Centered Research and Reviews, 5*(1), 28.

MacFarlane, A., Huschke, S., Pottie, K., Hauck, F.R., Griswold, K., and Harris, M.F. (2020). Barriers to the use of trained interpreters in consultations with refugees in four resettlement countries: A qualitative analysis using normalisation process theory. *BMC Family Practice, 21*, 1–8.

Miller, K.E., Martell, Z.L., Pazdirek, L., Caruth, M., and Lopez, D. (2005). The role of interpreters in psychotherapy with refugees: An exploratory study. *American Journal of Orthopsychiatry, 75*(1), 27–39.

Moser-Mercer, B., Qudah, S., Ali Malkawi, M.N., Mutiga, J., and Al-Batineh, M. (2021). Beyond aid: Sustainable responses to meeting language communication needs in humanitarian contexts. *Interpreting and Society, 1*(1), 5–27.

Pandey, M., Maina, R.G., Amoyaw, J., Li, Y., Kamrul, R., Michaels, C.R., and Maroof, R. (2021). Impacts of English language proficiency on healthcare access, use, and outcomes among immigrants: A qualitative study. *BMC Health Services Research, 21*, 1–13.

Rajiv, P., Riggs, E., Brown, S., Szwarc, J., and Yelland, J. (2021). Communication interventions to support people with limited English proficiency in healthcare: A systematic review. *Journal of Communication in Healthcare*, *14*(2), 176–187.

Rasi, S. (2020). Impact of language barriers on access to healthcare services by immigrant patients: A systematic review. *Asia Pacific Journal of Health Management*, *15*(1), 35–48.

Raval, H. (2003). Therapists' experiences of working with language interpreters. *International Journal of Mental Health*, *32*(2), 6–31.

Roat, C.E., Putsch, R., and Lucero, C. (1997). *Bridging the gap over the phone: A basic training for telephone interpreters serving medical settings*. Cross Cultural Health Care Program.

Sleptsova, M., Hofer, G., Morina, N., and Langewitz, W. (2014). The role of the health care interpreter in a clinical setting – A narrative review. *Journal of Community Health Nursing*, *31*(3), 167–184.

Tribe, R. and Morrissey, J. (2014). The refugee context and the role of interpreters. In R. Tribe and H. Raval (Eds), *Working with interpreters in mental health* (pp 198–218). Routledge.

UNHCR (2023). Operational data portal refugee situations: Uganda. Available at: https://data2.unhcr.org/en/country/uga (Accessed 16 December 2024).

UNHCR (2024). Uganda: Refugees and nationals by district. Available at: https://data.unhcr.org/en/country/uga (Accessed 23 May 2024).

WHO (2024). Uganda's Health System Addresses the Health Needs of Refugees, Migrants and Host Communities. Press release 25 March 2024. Available at: https://www.afro.who.int/countries/uganda/news/ugandas-health-system-addresses-health-needs-refugees-migrants-and-host-communities (Accessed 6 October 2025).

PART III

Programmatic organisation

SIX

Working for access: how Red Cross in Georgia works to ensure diagnostics and continuity of HIV care and treatment for Ukrainian refugees

Davron Mukhamadiev, Nana Tsanava, and Tea Chikviladze

This chapter discusses access to HIV services for people displaced by the crisis in Ukraine, focusing on the intervention by the International Federation of Red Cross and Red Crescent Societies (IFRC) and the Georgia Red Cross Society (GRCS). Over 245,000 refugees have arrived in Georgia since the conflict began, many facing significant barriers to healthcare, especially those living with HIV (PLHIV). Although Georgia offers free access to HIV services for persons registered as asylum seekers, refugees or persons with a humanitarian status, not all displaced Ukrainians have chosen to get registered to obtain a legal humanitarian status, and thus struggle to access essential services like antiretroviral therapy (ART). The IFRC/GRCS programme works to ensure continuous HIV care for this population, offering medical consultations, lab tests, and psychosocial support, supplementing state efforts. Key interventions included raising awareness, establishing communication channels, and collaborating with local health institutions. The findings highlight the need for uninterrupted HIV care, advocacy for rights-based healthcare, and solutions to integrate displaced populations into national health systems, focusing on reducing stigma and ensuring equitable access to HIV services.

Introduction

Contributing to the provision of basic health services for the most vulnerable displaced populations and addressing their urgent needs continue to be one of Red Cross and Red Crescent Societies top priorities. These priorities encompass maintaining the delivery of direct support to at-risk populations, enhancing advocacy to increase their access to health and care services (including those related to HIV), eliminating barriers, and progressing towards achieving UHC targets. Displaced people remain among the most vulnerable members of communities often faced with xenophobia; discrimination; poor living, housing, and working conditions; and inadequate access to health services, despite frequently experiencing physical and mental health problems.

Between 24 February 2022 and 15 February 2024, nearly 6.5 million refugees from Ukraine have been recorded worldwide (UNHCR collation of statistics made available by national authorities, 2024). Among these refugees, the majority (6 million or 93 per cent) were recorded in Europe (UNHCR, 2024). More than 60 per cent of whom are women and 35 per cent are children.

Since February 2022 more than 245,000 people from Ukraine have crossed the border into Georgia (Kajaia, 2024), of which approximately 29,000 have remained (UNHCR, 2025), many of them are from heavily war-affected areas in the east of Ukraine. It is estimated that between 0.16 per cent and 1 per cent of Ukrainian refugees live with HIV (ECDC, 2022).

While access to healthcare services was generally considered satisfactory for displaced people from Ukraine in Georgia, the findings of the 'Needs assessment of Ukrainian refugees in Georgia' (PIN, 2023) revealed specific challenges and barriers. Since April 2022, the Government of Georgia has issued several decrees, all of which aim to extend the state healthcare programmes to citizens of Ukraine who arrived in Georgia during the specified period and provide them with the same access to healthcare services as Georgian citizens. Despite these directives, numerous complaints have been reported to the GRCS by affected individuals and local municipalities regarding difficulties in accessing healthcare without identification. Additionally, healthcare providers have been requiring payment for services that should be provided free of charge under the Decree. This highlights the urgent need to ensure that both displaced individuals and healthcare providers in Georgia are informed about the rights and entitlements of those displaced from Ukraine. Additionally, it highlights the importance of enhancing risk communication and community engagement efforts aimed at displaced Ukrainians.

Access to HIV services for displaced persons from Ukraine presents a multifaceted challenge amid the backdrop of geopolitical tensions and humanitarian crises. Provision of essential healthcare services for people with HIV, especially access to ART underscores the imperative for comprehensive and equitable healthcare delivery systems.

The sociopolitical situation in Georgia affects the availability and accessibility of HIV services for displaced persons. Ongoing conflict in Ukraine has resulted in mass displacement in several countries. The displacement has increased the vulnerability of refugees living with HIV to stigma, discrimination, and violence, as arrival in new country, not speaking language, having no hosing and not being aware of the health system, especially in terms of access to the HIV services creates unfamiliar and unfriendly atmosphere, which may deter them from seeking or continuing ART (Parczewski et al, 2025).

The state health programme covers HIV services for Ukrainian citizens who have obtained, and been registered with a protection status (refugee, asylum seekers, humanitarian protection). Ukrainians who arrived in Georgia before February 2022, and thus did not arrive as refugees, cannot be included to the state programme.

According to the information from Infectious Diseases, AIDS and Clinical Immunology research Center (IDACRC) in Georgia, in total 125 foreign PLHIV from different countries: Ukraine, Russia, Belarus, Turkey, Iran, and Austria applied for treatment in 2023. These individuals receive ART free of charge, however IDACRC cannot provide regular medical services and accompaniment, including medical consultations and regular lab analyses, as they have not been registered as refugees, asylum seekers, or individuals with a humanitarian status. This lack of registration, which may be due to displaced people not considering Georgia as their final destination, or being reluctant to relinquish their passport, and thus future travel, with a humanitarian protection identification card, impacts their opportunities to access healthcare.

To address the needs of the most vulnerable people the International Federation of Red Cross and Red Crescent Societies jointly with Georgia Red Cross Society (2022–2024) launched the long-term comprehensive programme focused on assistance for vulnerable displaced people in receiving access to health services and social benefits on an equal basis with the local population. In this article, the primary outcomes of Georgia Red Cross interventions are ensuring better access for displaced people from Ukraine to HIV services in Georgia.

Programme design and implementation

To ensure effective and comprehensive programming, a series of priority tasks was outlined during the initial implementation phase. These tasks focused on understanding the healthcare needs of displaced people from Ukraine living with HIV in Georgia, as well as identifying key gaps and developing solutions to improve their access to critical services.

The prioritised tasks included:

- *Conducting a thorough needs assessment*: A deep and proper analysis of the barriers to healthcare access for displaced people from Ukraine living with HIV in Georgia. This included evaluating the specific needs of this vulnerable group and how they were affected by factors such as legal status, language, and other socio-economic conditions.
- *Analysing existing health services*: A comprehensive analysis of the current health services available for people living with HIV (PLHIV) in Georgia, with a particular focus on displaced people from Ukraine with varying legal statuses (for example, refugees, asylum seekers, people under humanitarian protection).
- *Identifying key support partners*: We identified and mapped the main partners providing health-related support to displaced people from Ukraine in Georgia, particularly those offering services free of charge, to facilitate access to healthcare.

The overarching strategy of our intervention was to enhance access to ART and other essential health services. We adopted a holistic approach that addresses not only the clinical but also the psychosocial, economic, and structural determinants of health affecting treatment adherence and healthcare outcomes for forcibly displaced Ukrainians in Georgia.

Protection as a cross-cutting issue

Our intervention was designed as an integral part of the broader protection framework, with a strong focus on ensuring safety, dignity, and meanisngful access to humanitarian aid. The International Federation of Red Cross and Red Crescent

Societies (IFRC) adhered to good programming practices rooted in the 'do no harm' principles. This meant prioritising the safety and dignity of displaced people, safeguarding meaningful access, and ensuring that all activities were accountable and participatory. Furthermore, we worked to enhance the social integration and adaptation of displaced people by providing access to critical health information and support services.

Collaboration and partner engagement

During the planning phase, IFRC and Georgia Red Cross staff organised a series of meetings with the IDACRC to gather comprehensive information on the existing medical services for people with HIV, with a particular focus on services available to the displaced Ukrainian population. These discussions gave rise to the following insights:

- *Health Service Access*: Citizens of Georgia, as well as individuals with officially recognised protection statuses (for example, refugees, asylum seekers, people under humanitarian protection), had full access to ART, including necessary health consultations, laboratory tests, and treatment regimens. This group of people consisted only max 10 per cent of the total number of displaced people. Meanwhile, displaced people from Ukraine without legal protection status (which makes up around 90 per cent of the total number of displaced people) faced significant barriers to accessing HIV-related healthcare services.
- *Antiretroviral Medicine Provision*: Medicines were provided free of charge by national health facilities, supported by the Country Coordination Mechanism (CCM) of the Global Fund for AIDS, Tuberculosis, and Malaria. This initiative covered all categories of people with HIV, regardless of their legal status.

Despite the availability of ART, two main gaps were identified:

- *Lack of Basic Healthcare Services for PLHIV*: A clear gap existed in the availability of essential health services for PLHIV, including regular medical consultations, laboratory testing to monitor viral load, and necessary adjustments to the treatment of people without any legal status. Without these services, effective and sustained ART was not possible.
- *Fear of Disclosure and Barriers to HIV Testing*: Many displaced people with HIV experienced significant fear and anxiety about disclosing their HIV-positive status, which created barriers to seeking HIV testing and treatment. This concern was particularly prevalent among those newly diagnosed with HIV, who were hesitant to access healthcare due to potential stigma or discrimination.

To overcome these challenges, IFRC and Georgia Red Cross established close, supportive relationships with local Ukrainian communities in Georgia, particularly in the three main areas where Ukrainians were living in concentrated communities: Tbilisi, Batumi, and Kutaisi. We facilitated confidential communication channels to ensure the safety and dignity of individuals seeking care. We also employed community-based outreach strategies by conducting informative and educational activities through the network of Georgia Red Cross volunteers, and in close collaboration with Ukrainian NGOs in Georgia, to promote the availability of HIV diagnosis and treatment, raise awareness, and disseminate critical information about available medical services. At the beginning of the provision of HIV services, GRCS received calls on the hotline with questions about the availability and access to HIV services, where and how to receive them, but later the calls were primarily requests to continue the support for HIV services, as it gave them a chance to access ART for free. The Georgia Red Cross Hotline service became one of the most effective instruments, and in most cases, the first point of contact for people living with HIV (PLHIV), where specially trained hotline experts could provide initial information on available health services and redirect them to more specific support from the relevant Red Cross or AIDS Centre experts. These initiatives aim to increase awareness and encourage individuals to seek necessary medical care.

Information dissemination and awareness-raising

As part of our awareness campaign, Georgia Red Cross, with support from IFRC, developed informational leaflets in both Ukrainian and Russian languages. These leaflets provided essential information about the available health services, including how to access medical assistance for HIV treatment, the importance of ART, and available support for those in need.

These informational materials were widely distributed through social media channels, shared with partner organisations, and placed at key points within the IDACRC, making them easily accessible to both displaced individuals and local healthcare providers.

Maintaining continuity and consistency in therapy was a key priority in this programme. Once a person with HIV was registered at the AIDS centre, communication with them was established through two interrelated communication channels:

- *Doctor–Patient Contact*: The assigned doctor maintains regular contact with the patient throughout the whole treatment period. Meetings occurred monthly, or more frequently if required, depending on the patient's health status and the results of their laboratory tests. If necessary, therapy adjustments were made based on the patient's condition.
- *Red Cross Support*: A social worker of the Georgia Red Cross conducts regular meetings with the patient, either face-to-face or online, to provide feedback on the treatment. During these meetings, the focus was on assessing whether any other factors were hindering treatment (such as financial issues)

and, when necessary, connecting the patient to additional assistance programmes (for example, for food, clothing, or vouchers).

The Red Cross social worker held regular coordination meetings with the doctors at the AIDS centre to receive updates and relevant information about the patient's progress. This system of continuous communication and support ensured that patients received comprehensive care and assistance throughout their treatment.

Considering the challenges and needs already discussed, between October 2023 and December 2024, a total of 102 (36.3 per cent F and 63.7 per cent M) PLHIV from Ukraine and countries affected by the Ukraine crisis registered by IDACRC were supported by the IFRC/Georgia Red Cross Society to access HIV services. At the time of joining the programme, all PLHIV were aware of their status and had a history of receiving ART in Ukraine. A small number of them arrived in Georgia with a supply of medicines, and most had a break in treatment from one to two months due to the problematic situation in southeastern Ukraine and the inability to access drugs at AIDS Centres. Many of them did not have documents in their possession, but they had information about their status, viral load, and remembered their ART regimens well.

Lessons learned

In total, 102 PLHIV from Ukraine and countries affected by the Ukraine crisis (Belarus, Russia) received HIV services through Red Cross. Red Cross covered costs for a monthly individual scheme of treatment: medical consultation and regular lab analyses. For one regular (mild) case, around 150–180 USD. ART medicines were provided free of charge by the IDACRC. In addition, the Red Cross covered costs for one severe case (min two weeks hospitalisation with complex treatment) at 1,800 USD per person, upon request of the IDACRC.

Throughout the entire period of supervision, the health status of the patients remained stable, and their viral loads remained suppressed. The Red Cross intervention contributes to improving the quality of life of people living with HIV, controlling the epidemic situation in the targeted population, and avoiding the spread of infection, mortality, and morbidity.

When HIV services were first offered, GRCS received calls on the hotline with questions about the availability and accessibility of HIV services, where and how to receive them, but later the calls were primarily requests to continue the support for HIV services, as it gave them a chance to access ART for free.

According to a manager at the IDACRC:

> The project provided an opportunity for the beneficiaries to receive not only a one-time service, but an opportunity for continuity/adherence/laboratory monitoring of antiretroviral therapy in dynamics. The Red Cross project was important at general as well as individual (patient) level. On one hand the patients had a hope that they will receive adequate medical services (free of charge) and on the other hand from the epidemiological point of view, the prevention of the spread of the disease was also present, as a person being on a treatment and with an undetectable viral load feels healthy and is not a source of infection for others.

Several critical factors emerged to significantly influence the continuity and sustainability of access to HIV-related services for displaced people from Ukraine. Our intervention demonstrated high demand for health assistance to PLHIV from Ukraine. It is essential to mention that, month by month, more and more people with HIV have started to apply to the Red Cross or AIDS centres to access these services. One of the most prominent challenges was the high mobility of displaced people from Ukraine. Many individuals frequently travel outside of Georgia, and in some cases, they leave the country entirely. This poses significant risks, particularly in terms of interruptions to ART and potential deterioration of their health over time. To mitigate these risks, it became essential to provide displaced people with guidance on how to maintain continuity of treatment, particularly advising them to reach out to Red Cross offices in infectious disease centres upon arrival in new countries. This ensures that individuals can receive the necessary support and continue their antiretroviral (ARV) therapy uninterrupted.

A major concern was the financial sustainability of the intervention and finding ways to ensure long-term assistance for displaced people from Ukraine living with HIV. The IFRC, in collaboration with the Georgia Red Cross, worked diligently to advocate for long-term solutions to address the ongoing needs of this vulnerable population. As part of this effort, IFRC/GRCS established and led a thematic health working group, which brought together a diverse range of stakeholders, including NGOs representing Ukrainian communities, representatives from AIDS centres, the Ministry of Health, and donor organisations. Unfortunately, despite these efforts, assistance remains highly dependent on international funding, with limited state support for these services. This dependency highlights the need for continued advocacy to secure sustainable, long-term funding solutions.

Discussion

The findings from this study highlight the significant barriers faced by displaced populations, particularly PLHIV, in accessing healthcare services and the critical importance of continuity of HIV care for PLHIV from Ukraine. The limited legal recognition of refugees and asylum seekers in Georgia has exacerbated the challenges of accessing HIV care. Many displaced individuals face uncertainty regarding their rights, especially in a context where access to HIV treatment and diagnostics is contingent upon meeting specific legal criteria. Krause et al (2000) emphasise the importance of integrating targeted health services, including reproductive and infectious disease care, within broader humanitarian interventions to enhance accessibility and improve health outcomes for refugees.

The Red Cross intervention in Georgia aligns with recommendations in the literature regarding the importance of integrating HIV care into broader humanitarian health programmes to ensure effectiveness and continuity of care for this population group. For example, calls have been made for healthcare systems to provide comprehensive, rights-based approaches to HIV care, ensuring that displaced individuals can access the services they need without facing additional legal or financial obstacles (Mendelsohn et al, 2014; Vasylyeva et al, 2022). The IFRC's programme appears to be an effective model for providing such services, addressing not only the immediate needs of PLHIV but also the broader structural barriers that hinder access to care, ensuring non-interrupted ART for displaced people from Ukraine during their stay in Georgia.

However, the challenges are far from over. While direct short- and mid-term interventions have proven effective, the long-term sustainability of such programmes and their continuity require addressing the underlying legal and social barriers. Reviews underscore the need for host countries to expand their healthcare systems to integrate displaced populations, including refugees with sexual health needs (Logie et al, 2024) and chronic conditions such as HIV (Brandenberger et al, 2019). Without such structural changes, displaced persons may continue to face uncertainty regarding their healthcare access, leading to gaps in treatment and increasing the risk of HIV transmission.

Conclusion

This chapter discusses the challenges faced by displaced individuals from Ukraine in accessing HIV services in

Georgia and evaluates the intervention provided by the IFRC and GRCS. The findings demonstrate that humanitarian interventions can effectively mitigate barriers to healthcare access, improving health outcomes for vulnerable populations. However, the need for a comprehensive and rights-based approach to healthcare for displaced persons remains critical. Legal restrictions, financial barriers, and lack of awareness continue to pose significant challenges to the full integration of displaced people into national health systems. Unfortunately, providing continuous therapy if PLHIV leaves Georgia permanently remains as a serious challenge. Now, no clear mechanisms for interaction between health systems of different countries have been developed, and in such a situation, IFRC and Georgia Red Cross recommend contacting the national Red Cross or Red Crescent Society for further recommendations on continuing treatment.

Long-term solutions must involve advocacy for policy changes that ensure universal access to healthcare, including HIV services, for all displaced individuals, regardless of their legal status. A crucial aspect of these solutions is the continuity of HIV care. Disrupted ART due to relocation or lack of consistent access to HIV medications and necessary medical services can lead to adverse health outcomes, including deterioration of health status and increased mortality. Ensuring uninterrupted HIV care should be a priority in any response to displacement, as it directly impacts the ability of individuals to live healthy lives. Continuous care involves not only regular access to antiretroviral therapy but also supportive humanitarian services that address the psychosocial and logistical barriers that displaced populations often face.

Additionally, fostering partnerships among international organisations, governments, and local communities will be key to addressing the structural challenges that hinder access to HIV care for displaced populations. In future, more sustainable solutions should focus on integrating displaced populations into the host country's healthcare system, advocating for the extension of rights to healthcare services, and reducing the stigma associated with HIV treatment. This will require a multi-sectoral approach that combines legal reform, advocacy, healthcare access, and education to promote inclusivity, equity, and solidarity in healthcare delivery for displaced people.

References

Brandenberger, J., Tylleskär, T., Sontag, K., Peterhans, B., and Ritz, N. (2019). A systematic literature review of reported challenges in health care delivery to migrants and refugees in high-income countries-the 3C model. *BMC Public Health*, *19*, 1–11.

ECDC (2022). *Operational Considerations for the Provision of the HIV Continuum of Care for Refugees From Ukraine in the EU/EEA*. European Centre for Disease Prevention Control. Available at: https://www.ecdc.europa.eu/en/publications-data/operational-considerations-provision-hiv-continuum-care-refugees-ukraine-eueea (Accessed 6 October 2025).

Kajaia, N. (2024). Microcredit helps Ukrainian refugees start businesses in Georgia. UNHCR. Available at: https://www.unhcr.org/news/stories/microcredit-helps-ukrainian-refugees-start-businesses-georgia (Accessed 30 May 2025).

Krause, S.K., Jones, R.K., and Purdin, S.J. (2000). Programmatic responses to refugees' reproductive health needs. *International Family Planning Perspectives*, *26*(4), 181–187.

Logie, C.H., MacKenzie, F., Malama, K., Lorimer, N., ... Perez-Brumer, A. (2024). Sexual and reproductive health among forcibly displaced persons in urban environments in low and middle-income countries: Scoping review findings. *Reproductive Health*, *21*(1), 51. doi:10.1186/s12978-024-01780-7

Mendelsohn, J.B., Spiegel, P., Schilperoord, M., Cornier, N., and Ross, D.A. (2014). Antiretroviral therapy for refugees and internally displaced persons: A call for equity. *PLoS Medicine*, *11*(6), e1001643.

Parczewski, M., Gökengin, D., Sullivan, A., de Amo, J., ... Rockstroh, J.K. (2025). Control of HIV across the WHO European region: Progress and remaining challenges. *The Lancet Regional Health – Europe*, *52*. doi:10.1016/j.lanepe.2025.101243

PIN (2023). Needs assessment: Ukrainian refugees in Georgia. People in Need. Available at: https://georgia.peopleinneed.net/media/publications/1832/file/pin-needs-assessment-report-ukrainian-refugees-in-georgia.pdf (Accessed 2 June 2025).

UNHCR (2025). Situation: Ukraine refugee situation. Available at: https://data.unhcr.org/en/situations/ukraine (Accessed 6 October 2025).

Vasylyeva, T.I., Horyniak, D.S., Bojorquez, I., and Pham, M.D. (2022). Left behind on the path to 90-90-90: Understanding and responding to HIV among displaced people. *Journal of the International AIDS Society*, *25*(11), e26031.

SEVEN

Working with mental health: how integrating mental health and psychosocial support into refugee health services can support continuity of care for chronic conditions

Ye Htut Oo

Refugees face substantial mental health problems throughout their migration cycle, which are linked to chronic disease conditions and protection issues they may encounter. Providing continuity of care for refugees with chronic diseases requires integrating mental health and psychosocial support (MHPSS) into the existing healthcare system. This chapter reviews the literature and guidelines on integrating MHPSS into existing healthcare services for refugees with chronic conditions to ensure continuity of care. Integration can be achieved at various stages of the healthcare spectrum, from promotion and prevention to treatment and rehabilitation, through scalable mental health interventions. MHPSS guidelines also provide essential principles, such as person-centred and community-based approaches, to deliver culturally appropriate physical and mental health services, ensuring continuity of care for refugees. Additionally, this chapter examines strategies for addressing the challenges of integrating MHPSS into existing health services for refugees with chronic conditions.

Introduction

Forcibly displaced refugees are individuals who have fled their countries because of traumatic experiences such as wars, conflicts and violence. They may face substantial mental health problems such as depression, post-traumatic stress disorder, psychosis and alcohol, and substance use conditions due to trauma experienced before migration, stress encountered during migration, and continued stressors after migration (Gagliardi, 2021). More than 1 out of 5 (22.1 per cent) people living in conflict areas have a mental health condition (Charlson et al, 2019) and the number is much higher than the global average (Fine et al, 2022). Of the more than 122 million people who are displaced globally, 87 per cent live in low- and middle-income countries (UNHCR, 2025), settings where mental health resources are limited (Silove, Ventevogel, and Rees, 2017). Such statistics emphasise substantial unmet needs of mental health services for forcibly displaced people.

In addition to mental health issues, the refugees are at increased risk for other chronic, non-communicable diseases such as diabetes and cardiovascular disease, and communicable diseases such as TB and HIV/AIDS due to poor living conditions, limited access to food, education, and healthcare (WHO, 2019). Mental health conditions and chronic diseases are closely linked to each other and share common risk factors such as biological, psychosocial, and environmental influences. For example, people who suffer from depression are more likely to develop cardiovascular disease, while patients with cardiovascular conditions are more likely to have comorbid depression (Li et al, 2023). Mental health problems are also linked with protection issues such as sexual violence, social stigma, or exclusion from education, healthcare, livelihood opportunities, or other services (UNHCR, 2019). These, in turn, create further obstacles for refugees in accessing mental health and chronic disease care.

To ensure care continuity for refugees, integrating MHPSS into existing health services is essential, as it helps address the complex and interconnected needs of refugees. Continuity of care involves coordinating healthcare coherently to address a patient's ongoing health needs, with the involvement of various healthcare providers and specialities when necessary (Meiqari et al, 2019). Integrating MHPSS can help mitigate the impact of mental health challenges on chronic disease management, and, conversely, address how chronic conditions can exacerbate mental health issues (IFRC, 2021). MHPSS refers to any local or external assistance aimed at enhancing psychosocial well-being or preventing and treating mental health disorders. It requires a collaborative approach across sectors, such as health, education, and protection, to ensure that humanitarian responses are safe and culturally appropriate. It also involves providing access to appropriate support for those with mental health or psychosocial issues, enabling them to care for their well-being (UNHCR, 2019).

This review examines the literature and guidelines on integrating MHPSS into post-migration health services to ensure continuity of care for refugees with chronic conditions. It also examines the challenges and barriers in implementing integrated care models and offers recommendations for their effective application in the post-migration health settings.

Integrating MHPSS into health services in refugee populations

In refugee settings, health systems generally operate in silos due to separate guidelines for care and providers trained to deliver specific forms of care, rather than integrated approaches for physical and mental health care. Funding mechanisms also contribute, as most funds from donors finance vertical and segmented programmes based on specific requirements and target populations. This fragmentation can hinder continuity of care, leaving refugees with chronic conditions vulnerable to poor health outcomes over time (IFRC, 2021). However, integrating MHPSS into the existing health services offers a promising solution for chronic disease care continuity. Continuity of care is a multidimensional concept that encompasses a trusting relationship between the patient and service provider over time (interpersonal and longitudinal continuity), effective coordination of care to ensure the patient's well-being (management continuity), and the availability of patient information across multiple providers (informational continuity) (WHO, 2018). The programmes which demonstrate different types of MHPSS integration follow, illustrating how mental health support enhances the continuity of care by addressing both physical and psychological needs simultaneously.

MHPSS can be integrated at various stages of care, ranging from promotion and prevention to treatment and rehabilitation, supporting continuous care throughout the patient's care pathway. The study conducted among Syrian refugees and Jordanians in Jordan integrated the MHPSS intervention into community-based health awareness and educational interventions. There were three groups in the study: those who received community-based health education sessions, those who received both community-based health education and mental health sessions and those who received standard care at clinics. The integrated mental health intervention showed much improved outcomes in cardiovascular disease (CVD) risk measures (including LDL, HDL, BMI, and HbA1c) compared to other groups at both 12 months and 18 months post interventions (Powell et al, 2021). Such integration of mental health support with chronic disease management demonstrates interpersonal and longitudinal continuity by promoting long-term engagement with patients and improving ongoing care outcomes.

Médecins Sans Frontières (MSF) also integrated mental health into NCD care model for Syrian refugees in Shantila camp of Lebanon. Psychologists provided mental health services through referrals from doctors or the patient support team. The study found that hypertensive and diabetic patients had twice the control compared to their enrolment status six months earlier (Kayali et al, 2019). This demonstrates that patients' clinical outcomes can be improved by incorporating the mental health component through coordination among different teams, ensuring both management and longitudinal continuity of care.

Another example is the integration of MHPSS into primary health care. In Bangladesh, the mhGAP-HIG training was provided to 62 health staff, including doctors, medical coordinators, and nurses, to integrate MHPSS services into primary healthcare in UNHCR-supported health facilities for Rohingya refugees. It was shown that nearly 1,200 mental health consultations were provided for the refugees, leading to a fourfold increase in mental health consultations within seven months. Moreover, the referral system from the community to camp-based facilities, and if necessary, to district hospitals, became functional (Tarannum et al, 2019). It illustrates management and informational continuity through the coordination of mental health services within the existing health systems to provide comprehensive care for refugees. Similarly, thousands of Syrian and Turkish doctors in primary health care settings received mhGAP training from 2016 to 2019 to address the needs of Syrian refugees in Turkey. The results showed that patients were highly satisfied with the quality of MHPSS services (Karaoğlan Kahiloğulları et al, 2020), indicating interpersonal continuity.

A comprehensive approach that integrates psychosocial interventions into their overall care can also improve continuity of care for refugees with chronic conditions. This includes cognitive-behavioural therapy (CBT), stress management techniques, and peer support groups to improve their well-being over time. A study of a modified CBT on patients with diabetes and comorbid depression in rural US showed that it improved both medication adherence and mental health symptoms compared to usual care (Cummings et al, 2019). In Zambia, a lay counsellor provided evidence-based counselling to individuals living with HIV, which reduced mental health symptoms and alcohol use, further illustrating the importance of integrated interventions for supporting continuous care (Kane et al, 2022). Similar interventions have been conducted on patients with hypertension and diabetes in Mae La refugee camp to improve the mental and behavioural health of the patients (ELHRA, 2005).

The Joint United Nations Programme on HIV/AIDS (UNAIDS) and World Health Organization provided ways to integrate MHPSS into the HIV service continuum, such as integrating individual and group psychological interventions with HIV prevention counselling, conducting HIV testing and post-test counselling with mental health and drug and alcohol use assessment, providing CBT for treatment adherence, and incorporating self-management and self-care through recovery and rehabilitation process (WHO, 2022). It was also mentioned that group support psychotherapy is a cost-effective treatment for depression in HIV patients, as it promotes well-being through coping skills and peer support (van der Heijden et al, 2017). Such integration provides continuity of care, covering the full spectrum of patients' health needs.

An increasing number of studies highlight the importance of integrating MHPSS into health services to enhance continuity of care for refugees. The International Committee of the Red Cross (ICRC) has developed a holistic, person-centred model to address the needs of individuals living with NCDs in humanitarian settings, particularly for Syrian refugees and vulnerable host populations in Lebanon. This model integrates NCD care, HIV treatment, MHPSS, and rehabilitation services through an internal and external coordinated referral system (Truppa et al, 2023), demonstrating how a multidisciplinary approach can ensure continuity of care for vulnerable populations. Similarly, Hémono et al (2018) suggested applying integrated, multidisciplinary, and human-centred care to fill the health needs of Syrian refugees in Greece. It highlights the need for coordinated care that addresses both physical and mental health domains over time to provide continuity of care for individuals with chronic conditions. Additionally, a high-level representative meeting among refugee-hosting countries on the Ukrainian crisis emphasised the importance of integrating MHPSS services into different health services to ensure sustainability (WHO, 2023).

MHPSS guidelines and conceptual foundation for the integration

The Inter-Agency Standing Committee (IASC) Guidelines on Mental Health and Psychosocial Support in Emergency Settings (IASC, 2007), the UNHCR Mental Health and Psychosocial Support Framework (UNHCR, 2019), and the Sphere Standards (Sphere Association, 2018) offer essential strategies for integrating MHPSS into sectors such as health, protection, and education. By providing minimum standards for planning, implementation, and coordination across sectors, they ensure a comprehensive approach to care that extends beyond immediate relief to long-term well-being. The WHO's mhGAP Humanitarian Intervention Guide (mhGAP-HIG) also offers practical guidance for non-specialised healthcare workers for integrating mental, neurological, and substance use disorders into general healthcare (WHO, 2015).

These MHPSS guidelines emphasise key principles such as 'do no harm', cultural sensitivity, trauma-informed care, and a rights-based approach. These principles ensure that MHPSS interventions are designed to avoid causing harm and meet the specific cultural and emotional needs of refugees. Understanding cultural perspectives in various aspects of MHPSS programming, such as assessment, hiring processes, information sharing, the provision of counselling, and feedback mechanisms, will help ensure that interventions are respectful, effective, and not harmful to the communities being served (IASC, 2007; Shah, 2012). For instance, to address the health needs of Syrian refugees, host countries must provide culturally sensitive services, such as avoiding stigmatising language and offering mental health awareness programmes, since stigma is deeply rooted in cultural beliefs (Woodward et al, 2024). These services help build trust between healthcare providers and refugees, facilitating interpersonal and longitudinal continuity.

A trauma-informed approach ensures that refugees feel safe, supported, and empowered to rebuild resilience, which can improve both mental and physical health outcomes (SAMSHA, 2014). The approach is applicable to sexual health screenings, such as testing for HIV, hepatitis B and C, and to handling patients who may have a prior history of sexual assault (Knights et al, 2022). Protecting human rights is also a fundamental principle. For instance, people with severe mental disorders or HIV patients are at higher risk of human rights violations and often face difficulties in caring for themselves and their families, have limited access to humanitarian aid, and are excluded from community participation. It is essential to make sure the services are non-discriminatory and inclusive, allowing vulnerable populations to fully participate in the programmes (WHO, 2015, 2021).

The guidelines also introduce a multilayered intervention pyramid, from basic services and community support to specialised care. This pyramid ensures management continuity by providing coordinated care at each level. At the community level, integrating mental health and chronic disease care within primary health services ensures interpersonal continuity, as providers develop ongoing, trusted relationships with refugees. The top layer of specialised services caters to severe cases, promoting informational continuity by ensuring that patient information is shared across providers to address both physical and mental health needs comprehensively. The guidelines also advocate for person-centred, community-based approaches that encourage active participation from refugees, families, and communities in managing their physical and mental health (Coulter and Oldham, 2016; IASC, 2019). This promotes both interpersonal and longitudinal continuity, empowering refugees to contribute to their own care and recovery, thereby building resilience over time.

Recommendations for overcoming challenges and effective implementation

There are numerous challenges in integrating MHPSS and chronic disease care in refugee settings. Structural issues, including government policies and sociopolitical factors, fragmented funding, organisational issues such as resource constraints and limited training of healthcare workers, and community-level issues like stigma and access to services, can pose significant challenges. Regarding the political constraint, Bangladesh, for example, is a non-signatory state to the 1951 Convention, and its related repatriation policy impacts the provision of humanitarian services to the Rohingya population (Khaled, 2021). In such cases, humanitarian organisations need to advocate for governments to make comprehensive policy changes that allow refugees to become self-reliant and access essential services. Another challenge is that funding is heavily reliant on donor interests, creating vertical programmes (Gyawali et al, 2021). It is recommended that donors be encouraged to adopt flexible funding models that integrate various services, rather than supporting short-term, issue-specific health programmes. Providing evidence on the cost-effectiveness and potential cost savings of integrated programmes, such as reduced duplication of services and improved health outcomes, will bolster support from donors for these long-term models. Building multi-sectoral partnerships to create more sustainable funding that covers a wide range of refugee needs is also essential.

In refugee settings, there is both a limited availability of trained professionals and scarce training opportunities for healthcare workers who can address both mental health and chronic disease care (Gyawali et al, 2021; Woodward et al, 2024). This is compounded by a lack of adequate research on integrated MHPSS models designed for refugees with chronic conditions. Using a community-based approach and training community members to provide basic mental health and support services, as well as scalable psychological interventions like Problem Management Plus (PM+) and 'Thinking Healthy', can help overcome these resource constraints. This task-shifting approach has been successful in reducing anxiety and depression, showing the power of peer support in helping others. By involving refugee community members, we can improve access to care, even when resources are limited (Cohen and Yaeger, 2021; Woodward et al, 2021). Creating a collaborative research initiative between humanitarian organisations, academic institutions, and local researchers is also crucial for providing evidence-based solutions for integrated healthcare models. A qualitative study among stakeholders in Lebanon, Uganda, and Indonesia prioritised 20 MHPSS research questions for humanitarian settings for 2021–2030. The topics closely related to chronic disease integration are No. 4 (integrating MHPSS into other sectors) and ranked No. 1 (strengthening the MHPSS workforce) (Tol et al, 2023). It is anticipated that solutions will emerge to address the shortage of trained professionals capable of providing both mental health and chronic disease care.

Another challenge is the financial and logistical constraints, which further limit the ability to provide comprehensive mental health and chronic disease services in these camps (Silove, 2021). More funding is needed to support both mental health and chronic disease care for refugees. By advocating for the mainstreaming of MHPSS in refugee aid services and increasing financial support, we can ensure that these critical services are available to serve the physical and psychosocial health needs of refugees. At the community level, stigma and discrimination surrounding mental health issues are extremely common (Xin, 2020), and there is also limited access to care, including medications (WHO, 2015, 2021). Thus, it is important to safeguard the protection of vulnerable populations by adopting a human rights-based approach. Innovative solutions such as mobile clinics and digital psychosocial interventions could increase refugees' access to much-needed services. Furthermore, language and cultural barriers are common in refugee programmes (Filmer et al, 2023). For instance, providing Westernised psychological assessments and counselling is not culturally appropriate for refugee settings of low- and middle-income countries (Amigues, 2022). Cultural considerations, a gender-sensitive approach, and faith-based models should be applied when programming integrated MHPSS interventions.

Conclusion

This chapter explains the significance of mental health and psychosocial issues in refugee settings and highlights their interconnectedness with chronic diseases. Responding to the needs of refugees with chronic physical and mental conditions requires multi-sectoral, collaborative approaches that are guided by guidelines such as the IASC MHPSS Guidelines, the Sphere Standards, and mhGAP-HIG. These guidelines provide a comprehensive, multilayered support system with underlying concepts and approaches, such as cultural sensitivity and a person-centred, community-based approach, to address the holistic aspects of well-being. Studies and projects on integrating MHPSS services into existing health services have demonstrated that this integration can occur at various stages of disease management, ranging from prevention to treatment to rehabilitation, resulting in improved health outcomes for refugees with chronic conditions. Despite challenges such as fragmented funding, limited resources, and social stigma, initiatives have shown successful outcomes when MHPSS is integrated into primary health care and community-based programmes.

It is essential to advocate for policy makers and donors to adopt an integrated approach, along with flexible funding models, to support the diverse health and psychosocial needs of refugees. A multi-sectoral approach, involving collaboration between governments, international and local organisations, as well as refugee communities, and coordination among different sectors of humanitarian organisations, is key to achieving sustainable solutions for the well-being of refugees. This teamwork will ensure that resources are utilised efficiently and that refugees are actively involved in decisions about their care. Additionally, scaling up evidence-based interventions, such as mhGAP and PM+, for healthcare workers in community-based approaches will be critical to overcoming resource constraints.

Integrating MHPSS and chronic disease care for refugees requires a combination of better policy changes, increased funding, effective training, and stronger collaboration. By developing an approach that addresses both mental and physical health needs in a coordinated way, we can improve refugees' well-being and ensure the long-term continuity of the comprehensive care they deserve.

References

Amigues, A. (2022). *Challenges and opportunities for culturally sensitive mental health and psychosocial support in the African context* (Masters). University of Uppsala. Available at: https://www.diva-portal.org/smash/get/diva2:1682389/FULLTEXT01.pdf (Accessed 27 August 2025).

Charlson, F., van Ommeren, M., Flaxman, A., Cornett, J., Whiteford, H., and Saxena, S. (2019). New WHO prevalence estimates of mental disorders in conflict settings: A systematic review and meta-analysis. *The Lancet*, *394*(10194), 240–248.

Cohen, F. and Yaeger, L. (2021). Task-shifting for refugee mental health and psychosocial support: A scoping review of services in humanitarian settings through the lens of RE-AIM. *Implementation Research and Practice*, *2*, 2633489521998790.

Coulter, A. and Oldham, J. (2016). Person-centred care: What is it and how do we get there? *Future Healthcare Journal*, *3*(2), 114–116.

Cummings, D.M., Lutes, L.D., Littlewood, K., Solar, C., ... Edwards, S. (2019). Randomized trial of a tailored cognitive behavioral intervention in type 2 diabetes with comorbid depressive and/or regimen-related distress symptoms: 12-month outcomes from COMRADE. *Diabetes Care*, *42*(5), 841–848.

ELRHA (2025). Integrating an evidence-based mental health intervention into non-communicable disease care. Available at: https://www.elrha.org/projects/integrating-an-evidence-based-mental-health-intervention-into-non-communicable-disease-care (Accessed 6 October 2025).

Filmer, T., Ray, R., and Glass, B.D. (2023). Barriers and facilitators experienced by migrants and refugees when accessing pharmaceutical care: A scoping review. *Research in Social and Administrative Pharmacy*, *19*, 977–988.

Fine, S.L., Kane, J.C., Spiegel, P.B., Tol, W.A., and Ventevogel, P. (2022). Ten years of tracking mental health in refugee primary health care settings: An updated analysis of data from UNHCR's Health Information System (2009–2018). *BMC Medicine*, *20*(1), 183.

Gagliardi, R. (2021). Traumatic situations and mental disorders in migrants, refugees and asylum seekers. *Psychiatry and Neuroscience Update: From Epistemology to Clinical Psychiatry*, *4*, 497–523.

Gyawali, B., Harasym, M.C., Hassan, S., Cooper, K., ... Tellier, S. (2021). Not an 'either/or': Integrating mental health and psychosocial support within non-communicable disease prevention and care in humanitarian response. *Journal of Global Health*, *11*, 03119.

Hémono, R., Relyea, B., Scott, J., Khaddaj, S., Douka, A., and Wringe, A. (2018). 'The needs have clearly evolved as time has gone on': A qualitative study to explore stakeholders' perspectives on the health needs of Syrian refugees in Greece following the 2016 European Union-Turkey agreement. *Conflict and Health*, *12*, 1–9.

IASC (2007). *IASC Guidelines on Mental Health and Psychosocial Support in Emergency Settings.* Inter-Agency Standing Committee. Available at: https://interagencystandingcommittee.org/iasc-task-force-mental-health-and-psychosocial-support-emergency-settings/iasc-guidelines-mental-health-and-psychosocial-support-emergency-settings-2007 (Accessed 2 June 2025).

IASC (2019). Community-based approaches to MHPSS programmes: A guidance note. Inter-Agency Standing Committee. Available at: https://interagencystandingcommittee.org/iasc-reference-group-mental-health-and-psychosocial-support-emergency-settings/iasc-community-based-approaches-mhpss-programmes-guidance-note (Accessed 2 June 2025).

IFRC (2021). *Integrating Mental Health and Psychosocial Support within Noncommunicable Disease Prevention and Care in Humanitarian Response: An exploratory review.* IFRC Reference Centre for Psychosocial Support.

Kane, J.C., Sharma, A., Murray, L.K., Chander, G., ... Cropsey, K. (2022). Efficacy of the common elements treatment approach (CETA) for unhealthy alcohol use among adults with HIV in Zambia: Results from a pilot randomized controlled trial. *AIDS and Behavior, 26*(2), 523–536.

Karaoğlan Kahiloğulları, A., Alataş, E., Ertuğrul, F., and Malaj, A. (2020). Responding to mental health needs of Syrian refugees in Turkey: mhGAP training impact assessment. *International Journal of Mental Health Systems, 14,* 1–9.

Kayali, M., Moussally, K., Lakis, C., Abrash, M.A., Sawan, C., Reid, A., and Edwards, J. (2019). Treating Syrian refugees with diabetes and hypertension in Shatila refugee camp, Lebanon: Médecins Sans Frontières model of care and treatment outcomes. *Conflict and Health, 13,* 1–11.

Khaled, A.F.M. (2021). Do no harm in refugee humanitarian aid: The case of the Rohingya humanitarian response. *Journal of International Humanitarian Action, 6*(1), 7.

Knights, F., Munir, S., Ahmed, H., and Hargreaves, S. (2022). Initial health assessments for newly arrived migrants, refugees, and asylum seekers. *BMJ, 377,* e068821.

Li, X., Zhou, J., Wang, M., Yang, C., and Sun, G. (2023). Cardiovascular disease and depression: A narrative review. *Frontiers in Cardiovascular Medicine*, *10*, 1274595.

Meiqari, L., Al-Oudat, T., Essink, D., Scheele, F., and Wright, P. (2019). How have researchers defined and used the concept of 'continuity of care' for chronic conditions in the context of resource-constrained settings? A scoping review of existing literature and a proposed conceptual framework. *Health Research Policy and Systems*, *17*, 1–14.

Powell, T.M., Li, S.-J., Hsiao, Y., Thompson, M., Farraj, A., Abdoh, M., and Farraj, R. (2021). An integrated physical and mental health awareness education intervention to reduce non-communicable diseases among Syrian refugees and Jordanians in host communities: A natural experiment study. *Preventive Medicine Reports*, *21*, 101310.

SAMSHA (2014). *SAMHSA's Concept of Trauma and Guidance for a Trauma-Informed Approach*. MF Substance Abuse and Mental Health Services Administration.

Shah, S.A. (2012). Ethical standards for transnational mental health and psychosocial support (MHPSS): Do no harm, preventing cross-cultural errors and inviting pushback. *Clinical Social Work Journal*, *40*, 438–449.

Silove, D. (2021). Challenges to mental health services for refugees: A global perspective. *World Psychiatry*, *20*(1), 131.

Silove, D., Ventevogel, P., and Rees, S. (2017). The contemporary refugee crisis: An overview of mental health challenges. *World Psychiatry*, *16*(2), 130–139.

Sphere Association (2018). *The Sphere Handbook: Humanitarian Charter and Minimum Standards in Humanitarian Response*. Sphere Association. Available at: www.spherestandards.org/handbook (Accessed 6 October 2025).

Tarannum, S., Elshazly, M., Harlass, S., and Ventevogel, P. (2019). Integrating mental health into primary health care in Rohingya refugee settings in Bangladesh: Experiences of UNHCR. *Intervention Journal of Mental Health and Psychosocial Support in Conflict Affected Areas*, *17*(2), 130–139.

Tol, W.A., Le, P.D., Harrison, S.L., Galappatti, A., ... Engels, M. (2023). Mental health and psychosocial support in humanitarian settings: Research priorities for 2021–30. *The Lancet Global Health*, *11*(6), e969–e975.

Truppa, C., Ansbro, É., Willis, R., Zmeter, C., ... Perel, P. (2023). Developing an integrated model of care for vulnerable populations living with non-communicable diseases in Lebanon: An online theory of change workshop. *Conflict and Health*, *17*(1), 35.

UNHCR (2019). Mental *health and psychosocial support*. Emergency Handbook. Available at: https://www.humanitarianlibrary.org/sites/default/files/2019/09/Emergency%20handbook_0.pdf (Accessed 6 October 2025).

UNHCR (2024). Mid-Year Trends 2024. UNHCR Global Data Service. Available at: https://www.unhcr.org/media/mid-year-trends-2024 (Accessed 6 October 2025).

van der Heijden, I., Abrahams, N., and Sinclair, D. (2017). Psychosocial group interventions to improve psychological well-being in adults living with HIV. Cochrane Database of Systematic Reviews, *14*(3), CD010806.

WHO (2015). mhGAP Humanitarian Intervention Guide (mhGAP-HIG): Clinical management of mental, neurological and substance use conditions in humanitarian emergencies. WHO. Available at: https://www.who.int/publications/i/item/9789241548922 (Accessed 2 June 2025).

WHO (2018). Continuity and coordination of care: A practice brief to support implementation of the WHO Framework on integrated people-centred health services. WHO. Available at: https://www.who.int/publications/i/item/9789241514033 (Accessed 2 June 2025).

WHO (2019). Migrants and refugees at higher risk of developing ill health than host populations, reveals first-ever WHO report on the health of displaced people in Europe. 2019. WHO. Available at: https://www.who.int/europe/news/item/21-01-2019-migrants-and-refugees-at-higher-risk-of-developing-ill-health-than-host-populations-reveals-first-ever-who-report-on-the-health-of-displaced-people-in-europe (Accessed 6 October 2025).

WHO (2021). Guidance on community mental health services: promoting person-centred and rights-based approaches. WHO. Available at: https://www.who.int/publications/i/item/9789240025707 (Accessed 2 June 2025).

WHO (2022). Integration of mental health and HIV interventions. WHO. Available at: https://www.who.int/publications/i/item/9789240043176 (Accessed 2 June 2025).

WHO (2023). Subregional high-level consultation: lessons learned and best practice sharing between refugee-hosting countries in the context of the Ukraine crisis, 18–19 April 2023, Bratislava. WHO Regional Office for Europe. Available at: https://www.who.int/europe/publications/i/item/WHO-EURO-2023-8000-47768-70507 (Accessed 2 June 2025).

Woodward, A., Dieleman, M.A., Sondorp, E., Roberts, B., ... Broerse, J.E. (2021). A system innovation perspective on the potential for scaling up new psychological interventions for refugees. *Intervention Journal of Mental Health and Psychosocial Support in Conflict Affected Areas*, *19*(1), 26–36.

Woodward, A., Fuhr, D.C., Barry, A.S., Balabanova, D., ... Ilkkursun, Z. (2024). Health system responsiveness to the mental health needs of Syrian refugees: Mixed-methods rapid appraisals in eight host countries in Europe and the Middle East. *Open Research Europe*, *3*, 14.

Xin, H. (2020). Addressing mental health stigmas among refugees: A narrative review from a socio-ecological perspective. *Universal Journal of Public Health*, *8*(2), 57–64.

EIGHT

Working across sectors: how multi-sectoral integration improves participation in mental health and psychosocial support interventions for refugees

Jacqueline Ntombizodwa Ndlovu

This chapter examines the challenges and solutions associated with delivering care in preventive mental health and psychosocial support (MHPSS) programmes for refugee populations in humanitarian settings. Psychological distress among refugees, exacerbated by pre-migration, migration, and post-migration stressors, requires sustained interventions to prevent more serious mental health conditions from developing. However, barriers such as stigma, economic pressures, and lack of integrated services often hinder long-term engagement. Using the Journey to Scale project in Uganda as a case study, this chapter examines the transformative potential of integrating mental health with other sectors to prevent disengagement from MHPSS interventions. By integrating mental health support within broader systems such as livelihoods, the SH+ 360 model used in the Journey to Scale project addresses both psychosocial and practical needs, facilitating engagement and sustainability. This chapter emphasises the importance of integrating interventions to ensure relevance through participatory approaches, thereby enhancing the overall continuity of MHPSS programmes in conflict-affected settings.

Introduction

Mental health is an essential component of well-being, particularly in humanitarian settings where individuals face high levels of distress due to displacement, uncertainty, and trauma. MHPSS refers to a broad range of interventions that aim to improve mental well-being, reduce distress, and strengthen coping strategies (Tol et al, 2015). However, in humanitarian contexts, distress is often linked to unmet basic needs such as housing, food, employment, and safety (Hagen-Zanker et al, 2022). This bidirectional relationship means that while addressing these socio-economic needs can help alleviate distress, unresolved psychological distress can also affect an individual's ability to engage in livelihood activities or access essential services (Jiménez-Solomon et al, 2024). This highlights the need for integrated approaches that simultaneously address mental health and broader social determinants of well-being.

A key distinction exists between interventions aimed at preventing the onset of clinical mental health conditions by addressing distress and those designed to treat existing clinical disorders. This chapter focuses on the former – continuity of care for MHPSS interventions that mitigate distress and prevent more serious conditions through integrated, multi-sectoral approaches. Specifically, it examines how multi-sectoral integration, defined as embedding mental health support within broader social, economic, and community-based systems, can enhance continued engagement in preventive MHPSS programmes. Using the Journey to Scale project (Leku et al, 2022) in Uganda as a case study, this chapter explores how integrating mental health services with other initiatives, such as livelihood support, addresses both psychological and practical needs, making interventions more accessible, relevant, and sustainable. I argue that this plays a central role in supporting the continuity of MHPSS care. Despite the clear need for mental health support, maintaining long-term engagement in MHPSS programmes in humanitarian settings remains challenging due to several factors. High turnover among trained healthcare providers, driven by the temporary nature of humanitarian work, disrupts programme continuity and affects sustained participation (Korff et al, 2015).

Additionally, the lack of culturally and socially relevant programmes often diminishes their appeal and effectiveness, reducing participant engagement over time (Dickson and Bangpan, 2018). Furthermore, in contexts marked by displacement, resource scarcity, and cultural stigma, individuals often struggle to remain involved in MHPSS programmes, despite their proven benefits (Greene et al, 2024). However, for populations whose lives are characterised by previous and/or ongoing instability and trauma, staying engaged in MHPSS services is essential for symptom management and improving quality of life (Epping-Jordan et al, 2016; Charlson et al, 2019).

Mental health challenges and needs in refugee populations

Refugee populations often experience mental health issues at significantly higher rates than the general population (Hameed et al, 2018). This disparity arises from pre-migration, migration, and post-migration stressors. Common conditions faced by affected populations include post-traumatic stress disorder (PTSD), depression, and anxiety. A comprehensive review by Blackmore and colleagues reported prevalence rates among refugees and asylum seekers as approximately 31.5 per cent for PTSD and depression, 11 per cent for anxiety disorders, and 1.5 per cent for psychosis (Blackmore et al, 2020). Furthermore, according to a study by Charlson and colleagues (2019), approximately 22 per cent of individuals in humanitarian settings suffer from some form of psychological distress, a figure that is likely conservative given the stigma and underreporting associated with mental health conditions in many cultures. The chronic nature of these conditions, often worsened by repeated trauma, necessitates a consistent and ongoing approach to mental health care.

The IASC has developed guidelines advocating for a multilayered approach to MHPSS in emergency settings (IASC, 2007). These guidelines are essential for ensuring continuity of care by providing a structured framework that addresses mental health and psychosocial needs across varying levels of severity and accessibility. This approach integrates four levels of intervention, ranging from basic services and community support to specialised mental health care, enabling individuals to transition between levels of need as their circumstances evolve. By promoting collaboration among healthcare providers, community workers, and specialised professionals, the guidelines reduce disruptions in care and facilitate a more cohesive support system. Additionally, the focus on contextually appropriate and scalable interventions ensures that MHPSS programmes remain effective even in resource-limited settings. Meanwhile, capacity-building initiatives help strengthen local systems for sustained care. Together, these elements support the development of an adaptable and coordinated MHPSS framework that prioritises the continuity and accessibility of care in humanitarian contexts.

However, while these guidelines offer a comprehensive framework, dropout rates from MHPSS programmes remain high, and despite coordinated and well-meaning efforts, continuity of care is not always achieved. In refugee populations where survival needs often take precedence, mental health care can seem less immediate or necessary. For many refugees, barriers such as economic pressures, cultural stigma, and the lack of integration between mental health services and other essential services create substantial obstacles to ongoing engagement.

Barriers to sustained engagement in mental health prevention programmes

Understanding why refugees disengage from MHPSS prevention programmes is essential for developing interventions that promote long-term participation, particularly from the perspective of refugees. Research highlights several key barriers to sustained engagement:

Economic pressures and competing priorities

Not surprisingly, refugees usually prioritise meeting basic survival needs, such as food, shelter and income, rather than mental health care, as the psychological distress they experience is closely linked to these survival needs. When their basic and financial needs are met, their psychological distress is often reduced. Economic insecurity is a significant barrier to engagement, with individuals more likely to abandon MHPSS programmes when their essential needs remain unmet. Epping-Jordan and colleagues (2016) emphasise that mental health services, if disconnected from these immediate priorities, are often perceived as irrelevant to daily survival, leading to low engagement rates.

Mental health stigma

In many cultures, mental disorders are highly stigmatised, discouraging individuals from seeking help due to fear of social exclusion. For refugees, particularly men, cultural perceptions of mental disorders as a sign of personal weakness or moral failing can be particularly limiting (Adaku et al, 2016). The stigma surrounding mental health remains widespread in many societies, hindering help-seeking behaviours and perpetuating a culture of shame associated with psychological well-being (Ahad et al, 2023). This stigma is often compounded by additional barriers refugees face, such as the trauma of displacement, the struggle for survival and the pressures of conforming to new societal expectations. For example, a study among Somali refugees revealed that many avoided mental health services due to fear of judgement, highlighting the importance of culturally sensitive approaches to normalise mental health care (Betancourt et al, 2020). When mental health services are framed to align with values and understanding of the context, they are more likely to be viewed as a form of support, reducing stigma and encouraging help-seeking behaviours.

Psychological distress

Continuous exposure to trauma and stress can lead to psychological distress, making it difficult for refugees to participate in structured mental health programmes, including prevention programmes. Feelings of isolation and the demands of adjusting to new environments further contribute to disengagement, with many delaying help as a coping mechanism (Miller and Rasmussen, 2017).

Mental health services that work in isolation from broader support systems, such as housing, employment, or education, are often perceived as irrelevant. This is not surprising, given the strong interlinking of psychological distress with basic needs. On one hand, experiencing distress due to unmet basic needs can be viewed as a normal human response to circumstances. On the other hand, refugees with clinical-level conditions, such as PTSD, for example, require specialised care that acknowledges the chronic nature of their conditions. Failure to integrate mental health services with broader support systems reinforces the perception that mental health care is disconnected from real-world concerns, which ultimately leads to lower participation rates (Patel et al, 2010). Recognising this distinction between distress arising from immediate survival challenges and persistent clinical conditions can help guide more effective, comprehensive care approaches.

Towards multi-sectoral integration for continuity of MHPSS care

Multi-sectoral integration offers a potential solution to the challenges mentioned by embedding mental health services within essential systems like education, livelihoods, and social protection (Ndlovu, Lind, et al, 2024). This approach has the potential to normalise mental health care, reduce stigma, and enhance relevance by addressing both psychological and practical needs. Linking MHPSS programmes with broader resilience-building initiatives such as economic empowerment, social support, and education can create more accessible, effective and sustainable mental health support systems by addressing both psychological and structural needs.

The SH+ programme: a case study in multi-sectoral integration

The Self-Help Plus (SH+) programme, developed by the WHO, provides an excellent example of multi-sectoral integration in practice (WHO, 2021). SH+ is a guided self-help intervention designed to help individuals in high-stress settings manage psychological distress. It is structured around audio recordings and an illustrated self-help book, guiding participants through exercises on mindfulness, acceptance, and problem-solving. This self-help approach minimises the need for professional mental health providers as briefly trained non-specialists deliver the service, making SH+ particularly suitable for low-resource settings, such as humanitarian settings (Epping-Jordan et al, 2016).

SH+ has been evaluated in multiple countries, including Uganda (Tol et al, 2020), Turkey (Acarturk et al, 2022), and five European countries (Purgato et al, 2021) to assess its effectiveness in managing stress and preventing mental disorders among refugees and asylum seekers. Randomised controlled trials in these settings showed SH+ significantly reduced psychological distress. These findings suggest that SH+ is a promising and scalable intervention for addressing mental health needs in diverse humanitarian contexts.

Building on this work, the Uganda research team further developed the SH+ programme into a model known as SH+ 360. This model is designed to provide holistic support by integrating mental health interventions with additional components, such as livelihoods, to address both psychological distress and socio-economic challenges (Leku et al, 2022). By addressing both psychological and material needs, SH+ 360 aims to make mental health services not only accessible but also directly relevant to the daily lives of refugees.

The SH+ 360 model was implemented through the Journey to Scale project, which sought to expand the reach of SH+ by integrating it into diverse humanitarian sectors in Uganda, including health, protection, and livelihoods (Ndlovu, Lind, et al, 2024). SH+ was integrated with two types of programming: one with BRAC Uganda, a financing-for-refugees project, and the other with the Safety, Protection, and Peaceful Coexistence (SPACE) project. As the projects were already ongoing, participants were familiar. They trusted BRAC Uganda and each other, and had already formed strong working groups, making it easier to integrate a mental health component, such as SH+, into these projects. The sense of familiarity contributed to continued engagement in care. In collaboration with the Ministry of Health, SH+ was integrated into their healthcare programming, providing psychosocial support to healthcare staff on the frontlines during the COVID-19 pandemic. With pandemic experiences still lingering, the need for a service such as SH+ was high and greatly needed by healthcare workers, thus leading to increased engagement with care.

The Journey to Scale project involved training intervention facilitators, adapting SH+ materials to local languages and contexts, and conducting needs assessments to identify barriers and facilitators to the implementation of SH+ 360 (Ndlovu, Ouizzane, et al, 2024). These efforts ensured that the programme was culturally appropriate and aligned with the needs of populations and partner organisations, facilitating engagement and uptake.

How SH+ 360 promotes engagement and continuity of care

Mental health interventions should be strategically integrated into broader sectoral programmes, including finance, income-generation, social protection, and other key development areas, to enhance engagement and ensure continuity of care. This approach recognises that mental well-being is deeply interconnected with economic stability, social security, and overall quality of life, and directly addresses the challenge of economic pressures and competing priorities. A practical example of such integration was demonstrated in our partnership with BRAC Uganda, where the SH+ was embedded within a financing and protection project through the SH+ 360 model (Ndlovu, Ouizzane et al, 2024). By linking mental health support with economic/livelihoods and safety and protection projects, participants gained access to a more holistic support system that simultaneously addressed multiple dimensions of their well-being. This integration allowed them to not only receive psychological support but also improve their financial security and social resilience, leading to better engagement and participation: 'There has been an improvement in attendance for savings (Income Generating Activity) because of integrating with the SH+ intervention, which could bring all the participants in the income generating activities together to attend the five-week training' (Partner staff, female, aged 29 years).

However, for such multi-sectoral integration interventions to be effectively implemented and scaled, the value of this approach must be communicated at various levels of influence.

Traditional funding models often operate in silos, focusing on singular aspects of development such as mental health, economic empowerment, or social protection. Engaging with funders and advocating for adaptable funding structures that recognise the added value of cross-sectoral approaches is essential to facilitate integrated interventions. Transforming these funding models will enable holistic and continuous care, ensuring that mental health is addressed in a comprehensive and integrated manner, rather than in isolation. Another level is the participants' level who are engaged in multi-sectoral interventions. For participants to fully benefit from integrated multi-sectoral interventions, they must understand the interconnectedness of the services they are engaged in. Clear communication about how mental health influences financial stability and social well-being can motivate individuals to actively engage in multiple programme components and maximise the benefits of participation.

> Without a person having a clear mind, they cannot handle anything given to them very well. They will not be able to keep the goats that you support them with, and even when you talk about protection, gender-based violence and so on, someone may not be able to handle them very well unless you support them with mental health and psychosocial support. (Partner staff, male, aged 42)

Programme implementers also play an essential role in effectively implementing integrated multi-sectoral interventions. Capacity strengthening efforts should equip them with the knowledge and skills necessary to deliver multi-sectoral programmes effectively. In the Journey to Scale project, we operationalised this practically by training partner staff in the implementation of SH+, so that when the project ended, they could continue delivering SH+ and continue training others as well to deliver SH+.

Cultural and contextual relevance is another cornerstone of SH+ 360. In the Journey to Scale project, the programme's materials were tailored to local languages and norms, ensuring relatability and fostering trust among participants. One participant noted: 'It is through these trainings that my home is at peace and that I am an important person to myself and the people around me' (Participant 021, male, aged 32).

By embedding the programme in culturally meaningful practices, SH+ 360 encourages participants to remain engaged.

Participation and ownership play a crucial role in ensuring continuity of care in MHPSS programmes, as they facilitate a sense of commitment, attachment, and accountability among participants. When individuals are actively involved in designing and implementing interventions, they develop a deeper connection to the programme, increasing the likelihood of sustained engagement. Results from the Journey to Scale project also highlighted the importance of inclusive and participatory approaches, particularly in keeping participants engaged and continuously attending sessions:

> The participatory part that was developed in the project, like making people take charge in the project, because when you involve people from the very beginning, people get attached to the project you are going to implement. You will find that the sustainability part of the project is well assured because the participatory part of it would ensure that people do not miss any part of the sessions when it comes to the intervention. (Participant 015, female, aged 34)

By involving participants from the outset, programmes become more responsive to their needs, creating a shared sense of ownership that promotes long-term success. This participatory approach not only ensures relevance but also builds trust and local capacity, making continuity of care more achievable, even in resource-constrained settings.

There is a strong bidirectional relationship between mental health and other social determinants of health, such as economic security, education, and social protection. Addressing these determinants in isolation limits the effectiveness of interventions. An integrated approach ensures that improvements in one area reinforce progress in other places, providing a more holistic manner of addressing people's challenges. For example, when mental health support is combined with livelihood initiatives, participants not only gain psychological resilience but also develop financial stability, which in turn further enhances their mental well-being. This interconnectedness has been observed by partners implementing SH+ 360 in the Journey to Scale project. One partner staff member noted how integrating mental health with livelihood activities in their project led to improved financial behaviours and stronger participation:

> Handling of money is not all that good but with the implementation of SH+ and its integration with the livelihood activities with these groups, you will find that women are more serious and even more focused within their saving groups, and only then (after the project) there is a great improvement when it comes to handling their Income Generating Activities. (Partner staff, female, aged 29)

This aligns with the broader observation that integrating services enhances participation and continued engagement in MHPSS programmes by addressing both the psychological and practical needs of participants, creating a more holistic and relevant support system. Multi-sectoral integration ensures that mental health care is not delivered in isolation but is incorporated into sectors such as livelihoods, education, and social protection, making interventions more meaningful and accessible. Participants in integrated programmes often experience immediate benefits such as increased financial stability, as highlighted by the earlier example, which further reinforces their commitment to mental health support. However, these benefits may not always be immediately visible, highlighting the need for sustained interventions that can be more long-term, as there are some gaps remaining:

> The SH+ was helpful because it has helped change many things regarding stress in my life. I can now handle stress when I experience it, and there is a difference now. However, stress is always there if there is nothing to help along with it, still, these sessions help at the moment, but if you have nothing, it still comes back. (Participant 001, female, aged 31)

SH+ 360 also builds community cohesion by maintaining the SH+ group-based delivery, which reduces isolation and strengthens social networks: 'The program has taught me a lot about relationships with people… it has helped me to learn how to stay with neighbours' (Participant 005, male, aged 55).

This sense of social connection, combined with the practical coping skills taught in the programme, empowers participants to manage stress and challenges more effectively: 'I was a victim of suicide because of overthinking … but through the skills I learnt, I can handle my problems and help my neighbours when they are overwhelmed' (Participant 013, male, aged 44).

The success of SH+ 360 is mirrored in other multi-sectoral MHPSS programmes. In conflict-affected settings like Iraq, the International Organisation for Migration's (IOM) MHPSS and Livelihood Integration project demonstrates the value of combining mental health and livelihood support (Duman et al, 2024). Participants reported improved emotional well-being, enhanced stress management, improved problem-solving skills, and stronger social connections, which fostered community cohesion and a sense of belonging (Duman et al, 2024). Addressing psychological and economic challenges, such integrated programmes enhance engagement and long-term sustainability. Similarly, evidence from other regions shows that embedding mental health services within broader resilience strategies increases retention and satisfaction. Programmes that align with participants' economic realities and cultural contexts offer tangible benefits, build trust, and encourage sustained participation, underscoring their transformative impact in conflict-affected communities. Studies show that participants in such programmes are more likely to advocate for the intervention within their communities, increasing its reach and impact (Greene et al, 2022).

Building on this evidence, several strategies are critical for preventing disengagement in MHPSS programmes. Holistic and relevant programme design that addresses mental health and socio-economic challenges demonstrates practical benefits, making sustained engagement easier for participants. Reducing stigma through community-based approaches, such as involving trusted local leaders as facilitators, enhances acceptance and participation. In the Journey to Scale project and broader SH+ work, SH+ is positioned as an empowerment and coping approach to deal with distress and adversity. This approach greatly helped in addressing and reducing stigma related to mental health. Additionally, integrating SH+ with other sectors that were identified as priority areas for participants also helped in reducing stigma connotations.

Engaging local leaders fosters cultural alignment and builds trust, particularly in communities where traditional approaches to mental health care may be met with scepticism. Offering flexible participation options and accommodating diverse schedules further improves accessibility and inclusivity. Finally, capacity building and sustainability planning are vital. Training community members to lead programmes builds local ownership and ensures continuity, even if external resources are withdrawn. In SH+ 360, facilitators emphasised the need for ongoing training to maintain high-quality delivery, while participants expressed a desire for further livelihood activities to prevent idleness and distress (Ndlovu, Ouizzane, et al, 2024).

The learnings from SH+ 360 demonstrate the value of integrating mental health care into broader support systems. By simultaneously addressing psychological, social, and economic needs, these approaches make MHPSS programmes more accessible, relevant, and sustainable. Investments in facilitator training, cultural adaptation, and livelihood integration will be crucial as humanitarian agencies seek to scale up such interventions. Sustained engagement depends on integrating mental health care within comprehensive systems that empower participants to rebuild their lives while meeting immediate needs, ultimately creating more impactful and participant-centred mental health interventions.

Conclusion

Multi-sectoral integration offers a promising solution for ensuring engagement and continuity of care in preventive MHPSS interventions. By integrating mental health services within broader support systems, models such as SH+ 360 make MHPSS interventions more relevant, acceptable, and potentially sustainable. Future MHPSS interventions that seek to increase participation, reach, and continuity of care should prioritise multi-sectoral integration, linking mental health with other priority sectors, such as livelihood, education, and social services.

References

Acarturk, C., Uygun, E., Ilkkursun, Z., Carswell, K., … Au, T. (2022). Effectiveness of a WHO Self-Help psychological intervention for preventing mental disorders among Syrian refugees in Turkey: A randomized controlled trial. *World Psychiatry*, *21*(1), 88–95.

Adaku, A., Okello, J., Lowry, B., Kane, J.C., Alderman, S., Musisi, S., and Tol, W. A. (2016). Mental health and psychosocial support for South Sudanese refugees in northern Uganda: A needs and resource assessment. *Conflict and Health*, *10*(1), 18.

Ahad, A.A., Sanchez-Gonzalez, M., and Junquera, P. (2023). Understanding and addressing mental health stigma across cultures for improving psychiatric care: A narrative review. *Cureus*, *15*(5).

Betancourt, T.S., Berent, J.M., Freeman, J., Frounfelker, R.L., ... Gautam, B. (2020). Family-based mental health promotion for Somali Bantu and Bhutanese refugees: Feasibility and acceptability trial. *Journal of Adolescent Health, 66*(3), 336–344.

Blackmore, R., Boyle, J.A., Fazel, M., Ranasinha, S., ... Gibson-Helm, M. (2020). The prevalence of mental illness in refugees and asylum seekers: A systematic review and meta-analysis. *PLoS Medicine, 17*(9), e1003337.

Charlson, F., van Ommeren, M., Flaxman, A., Cornett, J., Whiteford, H., and Saxena, S. (2019). New WHO prevalence estimates of mental disorders in conflict settings: A systematic review and meta-analysis. *The Lancet, 394*(10194), 240–248.

Dickson, K. and Bangpan, M. (2018). What are the barriers to, and facilitators of, implementing and receiving MHPSS programmes delivered to populations affected by humanitarian emergencies? A qualitative evidence synthesis. *Global Mental Health, 5*, e21.

Duman, Y., Meier, J., and Marzouk, H. (2024). Beyond survival: Transformative impacts of integrating mental health and livelihood support in conflict zones. *Journal of Peacebuilding & Development, 19*(2–3), 158–176.

Epping-Jordan, J.E., Harris, R., Brown, F.L., Carswell, K., ... van Ommeren, M. (2016). Self-Help Plus (SH+): A new WHO stress management package. *World Psychiatry, 15*(3), 295.

Greene, M.C., Bonz, A., Isaacs, R., Cristobal, M., ... Benavides, L. (2022). Community-based participatory design of a psychosocial intervention for migrant women in Ecuador and Panama. *SSM-Mental Health, 2*, 100152.

Greene, M.C., Wimer, G., Larrea, M., Jimenez, I.M., ... Demis, L. (2024). Strategies to improve the implementation and effectiveness of community-based psychosocial support interventions for displaced, migrant and host community women in Latin America. *Cambridge Prisms: Global Mental Health, 11*, e32.

Hagen-Zanker, J., Rubio, M.G., Lowe, C., and Mazzilli, C. (2022). *Basic needs and wellbeing in displacement settings: The role of humanitarian assistance and social protection*: ODI. Available at: https://odi.org/en/publications/basic-needs-and-wellbeing-in-displacement-settings-the-role-of-humanitarian-assistance-and-social-protection/ (Accessed 6 October 2025).

Hameed, S., Sadiq, A., and Din, A.U. (2018). The increased vulnerability of refugee population to mental health disorders. *Kansas Journal of Medicine*, *11*(1), 20.

IASC (2007). *IASC Guidelines on Mental Health and Psychosocial Support in Emergency Settings*. Inter-Agency Standing Committee. Available at: https://interagencystandingcommittee.org/iasc-task-force-mental-health-and-psychosocial-support-emergency-settings/iasc-guidelines-mental-health-and-psychosocial-support-emergency-settings-2007 (Accessed 2 June 2025).

Jiménez-Solomon, O., Garfinkel, I., Wall, M., and Wimer, C. (2024). When money and mental health problems pile up: The reciprocal relationship between income and psychological distress. *SSM-Population Health*, *25*, 101624.

Korff, V.P., Balbo, N., Mills, M., Heyse, L., and Wittek, R. (2015). The impact of humanitarian context conditions and individual characteristics on aid worker retention. *Disasters*, *39*(3), 522–545.

Leku, M.R., Ndlovu, J.N., Bourey, C., Aldridge, L.R., Upadhaya, N., Tol, W.A., and Augustinavicius, J.L. (2022). SH+ 360: Novel model for scaling up a mental health and psychosocial support programme in humanitarian settings. *BJPsych Open*, *8*(5), e147.

Miller, K.E. and Rasmussen, A. (2017). The mental health of civilians displaced by armed conflict: An ecological model of refugee distress. *Epidemiology and Psychiatric Sciences*, *26*(2), 129–138.

Ndlovu, J.N., Lind, J., Patlán, A.B., Upadhaya, N., ... Tol, W.A. (2024). Integration of psychological interventions in multi-sectoral humanitarian programmes: A systematic review. *BMC Health Services Research*, *24*(1), 1–18.

Ndlovu, J.N., Ouizzane, S., Leku, M.R., Okware, K.K., ... Tol, W.A. (2024). Scaling up mental health service provision through multisectoral integration: A qualitative analysis of factors shaping delivery and uptake among South Sudanese refugees and healthcare workers in Uganda. *Implementation Research and Practice*, 5, 26334895241288574.

Patel, V., Maj, M., Flisher, A.J., De Silva, M.J., ... Sanchez, M. (2010). Reducing the treatment gap for mental disorders: A WPA survey. *World Psychiatry*, 9(3), 169–176.

Purgato, M., Carswell, K., Tedeschi, F., Acarturk, C., ... Churchill, R. (2021). Effectiveness of self-help plus in preventing mental disorders in refugees and asylum seekers in Western Europe: A multinational randomized controlled trial. *Psychotherapy and Psychosomatics*, 90(6), 403–414.

Tol, W.A., Leku, M.R., Lakin, D.P., Carswell, K., ... García-Moreno, C. (2020). Guided self-help to reduce psychological distress in South Sudanese female refugees in Uganda: A cluster randomised trial. *The Lancet Global Health*, 8(2), e254–e263.

Tol, W.A., Purgato, M., Bass, J., Galappatti, A., and Eaton, W. (2015). Mental health and psychosocial support in humanitarian settings: A public mental health perspective. *Epidemiology and Psychiatric Sciences*, 24(6), 484–494.

WHO (2021). Self-Help Plus (SH+): A group-based stress management course for adults. WHO. Available at: https://www.who.int/publications/i/item/9789240035119 (Accessed 2 June 2025).

NINE

Working towards continuity of care: calls for action for forcibly displaced persons living with chronic illness

Lena Skovgaard Andersen and Morten Skovdal

The eight chapters in this volume demonstrate that continuity of care for forcibly displaced persons living with chronic illness is not the result of any single intervention, approach, or profession. Rather, it functions as an ecosystem composed of holistic care models, patient education, agency-driven approaches, community structures, translation and interpretation services, access facilitation, mental health integration, and multi-sectoral collaboration. Across the spheres of navigational capacity, social relations, and programmatic organisation, the chapters draw on diverse contexts – from Gaza to Georgia – to highlight practices that support equitable and sustained access to health services for displaced populations. Realising these practices at scale, however, requires concerted efforts at the macro level.

Political commitment is essential to embed refugee health within national strategies, legal frameworks, and health service entitlements. Displaced people, regardless of refugee status, must have guaranteed access to healthcare at every stage of the migratory pathway. Everyone has the right to the highest attainable standard of health. Without legal protections, continuity of chronic disease care is disrupted not because treatment is unavailable, but because systems are not configured to deliver services equitably.

Reliable and sustainable financing is equally crucial. Presently, chronic illnesses only make up a small proportion of the external aid for health. For instance, the WHO (2022) estimates that only 5 per cent of aid for health sent to lower and middle-income countries goes to addressing non-communicable diseases. Such underinvestment must be urgently addressed. When funding *is* made available, it must be flexible to respond to evolving needs on the ground and insulated from the constraints of short-term project cycles. Budgets must safeguard the supply of essential medicines, diagnostics, and human resources – from community health workers to trained interpreters – that make care possible.

Ongoing research is needed to build a robust evidence base that informs and strengthens context-sensitive practice. Participatory and inclusive research approaches can provide critical insights from those with lived experience, identifying barriers and facilitators to continued care, evaluating what works and can be scaled, and exposing what is failing and why. As emphasised in the WHO Global Research Agenda on Health and Migration (WHO, 2023), health responses to displacement must be data-driven. Knowledge cannot remain siloed in isolated project reports; it must be shared, tested, and refined across contexts.

Ensuring continued access to healthcare across the migratory pathway requires cross-sectoral collaboration and coordination. National governments, local healthcare providers, humanitarian organisations, local NGOs, researchers, host communities, and displaced populations must engage in equitable partnerships to address multi-level barriers and leverage facilitators.

Collaboration and coordination are a prerequisite for delivering uninterrupted care where continuity would otherwise be fragile.

Ultimately, translating the critical approaches highlighted in this volume into sustainable components of national and cross-border health systems depends on securing the macro-level enablers of political commitment, reliable financing, research investment, and effective cross-sectoral collaboration. When these foundations are in place, the initiatives proposed in these chapters can coalesce into a coherent and lasting response, ensuring that continuity of chronic disease care for displaced populations is not the exception, but the standard – anchored in equity, dignity, and the fundamental right to health (Aljadeeah et al, 2025).

References

Aljadeeah, S., Sy, H., Michielsen, J., Van De Konijnenburg, C., Ebadu, J.D., Procureur, F., and Heine, M. (2025). Access to medicines and continuity of non-communicable diseases care for forcibly displaced populations: A call for rights-based, comprehensive responses. *BMC Global and Public Health*, 3(1), 49.

WHO (2022). Invisible numbers: The true extent of noncommunicable diseases and what to do about them. WHO.

WHO (2023). Global research agenda on health, migration and displacement: Strengthening research and translating research priorities into policy and practice. WHO.

Index

A

accuracy of interpretation
 doubt about 85–86
 and workload 90–91
acquired immunodeficiency syndrome (AIDS) 39
 see also HIV
adherence to treatment
 and language barriers 79
 role of CHWs in monitoring 67–68
 see also medication adherence
Anderberg, Emilie Mai 4–5
antiretroviral therapy (ART) 38–39, 42–48, 103, 105–115
asthma 18

B

Babagoli, M.A. 70
Bangladesh, integration of MHPSS into health services in 122, 126
bias concerns, about interpreters 88
Bidibidi *see* cardio-metabolic disease care, role of CHWs in
Blackmore, R. 137
body mass index (BMI) 15, 25, 28
BRAC Uganda 142, 143
Braun, V. 61

C

capacity building 32, 138, 148
cardio-metabolic disease care, role of CHWs in 6, 58
 challenges 69–70
 community sensitisation and mobilisation 68–69
 delivery of prescribed medications 67
 health promotion and education 65–66
 monitoring of treatment adherence 67–68
 recording and examining conditions in community 68
 referral to health centre 64–65, 66
 relations between healthcare workers and community 61–63, 70
 screening and monitoring 63–64
 study 60–61
cardiovascular disease (CVD) 119, 121
caregivers, role in patient education 34
Charlson, F. 138
Checkpoint (community-based clinic) 47
chronic obstructive pulmonary disease 18
Clarke, V. 61
cognitive-behavioural therapy (CBT) 123
Collinsworth, A.W. 59
communication 31, 109
 interpreter *see* interpreters
 between patients and healthcare workers, role of CHWs in facilitating 61

INDEX

of refugees of healthcare professionals 47, 48, 50
with refugees with HIV in Georgia 110–111
community
  education programmes based on 29
  engagement, role of CHWs in 68–69, 71
  free clinics 47
  health education based on 121
  and healthcare workers, relations between 61–63, 70
  members, training of 127, 148
  and multi-sectoral integration programmes 147, 148
  outreach based on 32, 109
community health workers (CHWs) 29, 70–73
  as advocates for patients 62
  diverse roles of 72
  as intermediaries 61–62, 63, 72
  role in health-enabling community engagement 71
  special efforts of 72
  as translators 61
  in Uganda 59
  see also cardio-metabolic disease care, role of CHWs in
confidentiality issues, in interpreter-mediated communication 86–87
consultation time, and interpretation 89–90
counselling
  by CHWs 65, 66, 67
  and cultural sensitivity 128
  evidence-based 123
  for Gaza refugees about diabetes management 20, 22, 25, 27
  mental health 34, 35
  skills, of interpreters 95
Country Coordination Mechanism (CCM) 108
cross-sectoral collaboration 120, 127, 129, 154–155
  see also multi-sectoral integration
cultural sensitivity 20, 30, 32, 124–125, 128, 140

culturally tailored education 26, 29–30, 32, 33

D

Denmark, HIV care for Ukrainian refugees fleeing to 3, 4–5, 37–40
  arrival and integration phase 45–48, 50
  communication challenges 47–48
  health literacy 48
  and HIV-related stigma 44–45, 50
  humanitarian responses 45, 49–50
  informal alternatives 47
  insights from refugees 40–41
  pre-migration planning and preparedness 42–43, 49
  pre-war situation 39
  transit phase 43–45, 49–50
diabetes 3
  care, beliefs and attitudes towards 19–20, 32
  culturally tailored education for management of 26
  Gaza refugees *see* Gaza refugees, diabetes education initiatives
  management of 16
  neglect of care in humanitarian crises 16
  prevalence of 18
  see also cardio-metabolic disease care, role of CHWs in
digital psychosocial interventions 128
do no harm principle 108, 124
Dræbel, Tania Aase 6
duration of interpretation 85–86

E

economic pressures of refugees 139
emergency preparedness plans 17
Epping-Jordan, J.E. 139
evidence-based counselling 123

F

family
  and CHWs 61, 63, 70
  role in patient education 34

financial stability of refugees 139, 143, 144, 146
follow-up
 by CHWs 64, 66, 67–68, 69
 Gaza refugees 31, 32
 and patient education 34
funding 73, 154
 for HIV care 113
 integration of MHPSS into health services 126, 127
 mechanisms, fragmentation of 120–121
 multi-sectoral integration 144

G

Gaza refugees, diabetes education initiatives 4, 15–16
 baseline characteristics of participants 23–24
 counselling 22, 25, 27
 cultural and social barriers 32
 culturally tailored education 29–30, 32, 33
 educational intervention strategies 21–22
 follow-up care 31, 32
 glycaemic control 17–18, 19, 23–24, 25–27, 28
 limited resources and accessibility 31–32
 medication adherence 17–18, 19, 24, 25–26, 27
 mental health support 26, 29, 30
 overweight/obese patients 25, 27, 28
 patient engagement and motivation 32
 post-intervention improvements in HbA1c levels 24–25, 26
 recommendations for future education initiatives 33–35
 study 20–23
 sustainability of intervention 32
gender of interpreters 87, 93–94, 97
Georgia, HIV care for Ukrainian refugees in 7–8, 103–106
 access to healthcare services 105, 108, 111, 112, 113–114
 antiretroviral medicine provision 108
 collaboration and partner engagement 108–110
 costs of treatment 111
 fear of disclosure and barriers to HIV testing 109
 financial sustainability 113
 information dissemination and awareness-raising 110–111
 integration of HIV care into humanitarian health programmes 114
 lack of basic healthcare services 109
 mobility of displaced people 112–113
 priority tasks 106–107
 programme design and implementation 106–111
 protection framework 107–108
Georgia Red Cross Society (GRCS) 103, 105, 106, 108, 109–112, 113, 115
Global Fund for AIDS, Tuberculosis, and Malaria 108
glycaemic control
 and body mass index 25, 28
 of Gaza refugees with diabetes 17–18, 19, 23–24, 25–27, 28
 and medication adherence 25, 27
Greece, integration of MHPSS into health services in 124
group sessions, diabetes education 21
group support psychotherapy 123
Guidelines on Mental Health and Psychosocial Support in Emergency Settings, IASC 124, 138

H

HbA1c levels 22–23, 24–25, 26, 27, 28
health education, 4, 5, 48
 community-based 121

INDEX

role of CHWs in 65–66, 70
see also Gaza refugees, diabetes education initiatives; patient education
health promotion, role of CHWs in 65–66, 70, 71
health working groups 113
healthcare costs 7, 19
Hémono, R. 124
HIV
  antiretroviral therapy 38–39, 42–48, 103, 105–115
  Ukrainian refugees with *see* Denmark, HIV care for Ukrainian refugees fleeing to; Georgia, HIV care for Ukrainian refugees in
  service, integrate MHPSS into 123
  stigma related to 44–45, 50
Htut Oo, Ye 8
human rights, protection of 125, 128

I

Infectious Diseases, AIDS and Clinical Immunology research Center (IDACRC) 106, 108, 110, 111, 112
informational continuity of care 121, 122, 125
Inter-Agency Standing Committee (IASC) 124, 138
intermediaries, CHWs as 61–62, 63, 72
International Committee of the Red Cross (ICRC) 123
International Federation of Red Cross and Red Crescent Societies (IFRC) 103, 104, 106, 107–108, 109, 110, 111, 113, 114, 115
International Organisation for Migration (IOM) 147
interpersonal continuity of care 121, 122, 125, 126
interpreters
  balancing gender during selection 93–94, 97
  bias concerns 88
  confidentiality and trust concerns 86–87
  increasing the number of 93, 97
  mentorship of 91–93, 95
  multifaceted roles of 80
  multilingual, recruitment of 93–94
  patients' role expectations of 96–97
  teaching medical terminologies to 92
  training of 92–93, 95
  unprofessional conduct 91
  workload of 90–91, 97
interpreter-mediated patient-provider communication 6–7, 78–81
  accuracy of interpretation 85–86
  increased consultation and patient waiting time 89–90
  knowledge and skills needed for 94–95
  limitations of 80, 85–91, 94
  misrepresentation of information 88–89
  optimisation of 91–94
  provider-interpreter mutual expectations 96
  study 81–85
  training of healthcare providers 95–96

J

Joint United Nations Programme on HIV/AIDS 123
Jordan, integration of MHPSS into health services in 121
Journey to Scale project 135–136, 137, 142–143, 144–145, 146, 148

K

Kehlenbrink, S. 16
Khatri, R. 71
Krause, S.K. 114

L

language
  barriers 79, 80, 128

proficiency, of CHWs 61
training, for healthcare
    providers 95–96
see also interpreter-mediated
    patient-provider
    communication
Lebanon, integration of MHPSS
    into health services
    in 122, 123
longitudinal continuity of
    care 121, 122, 125, 126
Lubbad, Usama 4, 5
Lyles, E. 18

M

Mae La refugee camp,
    Thailand 123
management continuity of
    care 121, 122, 125
Médecins Sans Frontières
    (MSF) 122
medications
  adherence, 17–18, 19, 24,
    25–26, 27, 123
  HIV 38–39, 42–48, 103,
    105–115
  role of CHWs in 66–67
mental health 3
  counselling 34, 35
  issues, refugees with 119–120,
    137–139
  and social determinants of
    health 145–146
  stigma surrounding 125, 127–128,
    138, 139–140, 148
  support, integration into
    patient education 26, 29, 30,
    34, 35
mental health and psychosocial
    support (MHPSS) 135–136
  barriers to sustained engagement
    in 139–141
  dropout rates 138
  economic pressures and
    competing priorities 139
  mental health stigma 139–140
  multilayered intervention
    pyramid 125, 138

multi-sectoral integration 8,
    136–137, 141–149
  programmes, participation/
    ownership in 145
  psychological distress 135, 136,
    138, 139, 140–141
  strategies for preventing
    disengagement 148
mental health and psychosocial
    support (MHPSS), integration
    into health services 8,
    118–120, 120–124
  funding 126, 127
  guidelines and conceptual
    foundation for 124–126
  overcoming challenges
    and effective
    implementation 126–128
  political constraints 126
  protection of human
    rights 125, 128
  research 127
  resource constraints 126–127
  siloed nature of health
    systems 120–121
  training 126–127
mentorship of interpreters 91–93, 95
mhGAP Humanitarian
    Intervention Guide
    (mhGAP-HIG) 122, 124
MHPSS and Livelihood
    Integration project 147
misrepresentation of information
    by interpreters 88–89
mobile health clinics 32, 128
mobilisation, community 68–69
monitoring, role of CHWs in
    63–64, 67–68
motivation 32, 37, 42–43, 44,
    45–48, 49, 50
Mukhamadiev, Davron 7
multidisciplinary approach
  patient education 34
  workshops 22
multilingual interpreters,
    recruitment of 93–94
multi-sectoral integration 8,
    136–137, 141
  benefits of 146–147

INDEX

cultural and contextual relevance 144–145
funding 144
participants' understanding about 144
SH+ (Self-Help Plus) programme 141–143
SH+ 360 model 142, 143–149
Murphy, J.P. 71

N

Nakanjako, Rita 6–7
Ndlovu, Jacqueline Ntombizodwa 8
negotiators, CHWs as 63
Ngcobo, S. 71
non-communicable diseases (NCDs) 58, 59, 87, 119, 122, 123

O

obesity, and diabetes 25, 27, 28
one-on-one meetings, for diabetes education 21
online HIV groups 46

P

patient beliefs and attitudes towards diabetes care 19–20, 32
patient education 16
  community-based education programmes 29
  continuous follow-up and support 34
  culturally tailored education 33
  Gaza refugees *see* Gaza refugees, diabetes education initiatives
  integration of mental health support into 26, 29, 30, 31, 34
  multidisciplinary approach 34
  role of family and caregivers in 34
  and technology 34–35
patient waiting time, and interpretation 89–90
patient-centred care 9, 26, 30

patient-provider communication *see* interpreters
patient-provider relationship 6, 31, 96, 121
peer support 123, 127
Perry, S. 72
person-centred care 48, 125
political commitment, and continuity of care 153–154
Problem Management Plus (PM+) 127
psychological distress of refugees 135, 136, 138, 139, 140–141
  see also SH+ (Self-Help Plus) programme
psychosocial support *see* mental health and psychosocial support (MHPSS)

R

rapport of interpreters with patients 92
Red Cross *see* Georgia, HIV care for Ukrainian refugees in
referrals, role of CHWs in 64–65, 66
remote education 28
rights-based healthcare 105, 114, 115, 125, 128
Rohingya refugees 122, 125

S

SABRA healthcare centre *see* Gaza refugees, diabetes education initiatives
Safety, Protection, and Peaceful Coexistence (SPACE) project 142
screening, role of CHWs in 63–64
sensitisation, community 68–69
SH+ (Self-Help Plus) programme 141–143, 148
SH+ 360 model 142–149
social determinants of health 71, 145–146
social media 21, 28, 34
social practice theory 3, 9

social workers 47, 110–111
soft skills of interpreters 89, 95
Sphere Standards 124
stigma 125
  diabetes-related 32
  HIV-related 42, 44–45, 50, 105, 109
  medical conditions, and interpretation 86–87
  surrounding mental health conditions 125, 127–128, 138, 139–140, 148
Syrian refugees, medication interruption for 19

T

task-shifting approach for refugee MHPSS 127
technology, in patient education 34–35
telehealth 29
telemedicine 34
Thailand, integration of MHPSS into health services in 123
Thinking Healthy 127
training
  of CHWs 70
  of community members 127, 148
  of healthcare providers 32, 95–96
  and integration of MHPSS into health services 126–127
  of interpreters 92–93, 95
  mhGAP Humanitarian Intervention Guide 122
  of staff, in SH+ implementation 144
translation *see* interpreters
trauma-informed care 124, 125
trust 31, 50, 145
  and community-based approaches 148
  and cultural sensitivity 125
  in interpreters 80, 86–87, 97
  between patients and providers 96
  role of CHWs in building 70, 71
Turkey, integration of MHPSS into health services in 122

U

Uganda
  interpreter-mediated patient-provider communication in 6–7, 81–97
  Journey to Scale project 135–136, 137, 142–143, 144–145, 146, 148
  non-communicable diseases in 58
  Bidibidi *see* cardio-metabolic disease care, role of CHWs in
  SH+ 360 model 142–149
  Village Health Team programme 58–59
Ukrainian refugees, HIV care for *see* Denmark, HIV care for Ukrainian refugees fleeing to; Georgia, HIV care for Ukrainian refugees in
UNHCR Mental Health and Psychosocial Support Framework 124
United Nations Relief and Works Agency for Palestine Refugees in the Near East (UNRWA) 17, 20, 22, 29
United States, integration of MHPSS into health services in 123
unprofessional conduct of interpreters 91

V

Village Health Team programme, Uganda 58–59

W

workload of interpreters 90–91, 97
World Health Organization (WHO) 123, 141, 154

Z

Zambia, integration of MHPSS into health services in 123

www.ingramcontent.com/pod-product-compliance
Lightning Source LLC
Chambersburg PA
CBHW071708020426
42333CB00017B/2183